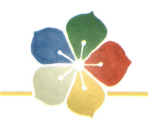

Welcome to Taste of Herbs!

This book contains all the recipes and remedies found inside the Taste of Herbs course. I thought providing this book would be a little easier than you having to print every PDF inside the website.

Please don't think of this as a normal book. Most books are meant to be passively read, absorbed, and filed on your bookshelf. Because of this, I prefer to think of what you are holding in your hands, as more of an invitation than a book.

Many people seeking information today spend a lot of time passively learning facts. But while facts may give you knowledge, they will never bring you wisdom.

Furthermore, when you simply learn facts, you will soon get caught up in the never ending amount of discrepancies of herbalism. As Rosemary Gladstar is fond of saying, "The only thing herbalists agree on is NOT to use aluminum pots."

The Taste of Herbs Course and this course exercise book are a remedy to memorizing long lists of facts. You learn by DOING, rather than passively reading.

Of course, you could just simply watch all the videos within the Taste of Herbs course as well as read the bonus monographs and ebooks. However, you would be missing out on the most crucial part of the course, which are the exercises you hold in your hands. I hope you accept this invitation to get in your kitchen, so you may dive deep into your personal herbal experiences.

Let's get started!

Rosalee de la Forêt

P.S. Remember to take Taste of Herbs one lesson at a time. Watch a short video, choose an exercise from this book, and move on to the next lesson. You will journey around the Flavor Wheel many times, learning more with each video lesson you watch and every recipe you prepare.

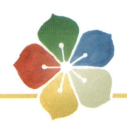

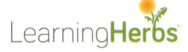

Taste of Herbs: The Complete Exercise Collection

by Rosalee de la Forêt.

©2015 LearningHerbs.com, LLC. All rights reserved.

No part of this publication may be reproduced in whole or in part, or stored in a retrieval system, or transmitted in any form or by any means, electronic, mechanical, photocopying, recording, or otherwise, without written permission of the publisher.

The herbal and plant information in Taste of Herbs and the *Taste of Herbs: The Complete Exercise Collection* is for educational purposes only. The information within the *Taste of Herbs: The Complete Exercise Collection* is not intended as a substitute for the advice provided by your physician or other medical professional. If you have or suspect that you have a serious health problem, promptly contact your health care provider. Always consult with a health care practitioner before using any herbal remedy or food, especially if pregnant, nursing, or have a medical condition.

Published by LearningHerbs.com, LLC, Shelton, WA

LearningHerbs, Taste Of Herbs, The Taste of Herbs Flavor Wheel, and associated logos are trademarks and/or registered trademarks of LearningHerbs.com, LLC. All rights reserved.

ISBN: 978-1-938419-54-6

First print edition, October 2015

Published in the United States of America

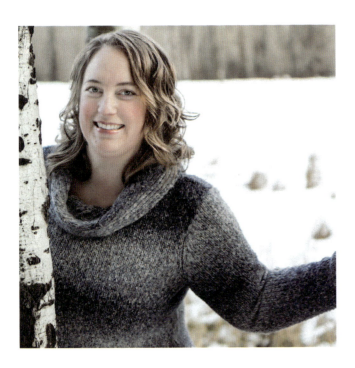

Rosalee de la Forêt is passionate about helping people discover the world of herbalism and natural health. As an herbal consultant, she helps people find natural solutions to their chronic health problems through her programs at HerbsWithRosalee.com.

Rosalee also teaches extensively about herbalism internationally and through her work as Education Director of LearningHerbs. She is the author of many articles, ebooks and courses about natural health and herbalism, including the T*aste of Herbs* course.

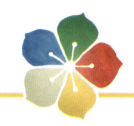
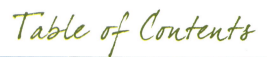

Table of Contents

Why is the taste of herbs important?....................5
The Five Tastes..11
Tips for Tasting Herbs.....................................12

Pungent..13
Introduction to Pungent
  Exercise 1: Discovering Diffusive Herbs...........14
  Exercise 2: Fresh Ginger vs. Dried Ginger.......15
  Exercise 3: Tasting Ginger.............................16
  Exercise 4: Tincture vs. Tea...........................17
Anodyne
  Cayenne Salve...18
  Basic Camphor and Menthol Pain Salve..........19
Antimicrobial
  Bee Balm Oxymel...20
  Cold Sore Lip Balm......................................23
  Vinegar Cleaner..24
Antispasmodic
  Antispasmodic liniment.................................26
  Cramp bark Chai...27
Anxiolytic
  Kava Hot Cocoa..28
Aphrodisiac
  Cardamom and Chia Seed Pudding................30
  Damiana Tea..31
  Sexy Chai Blend..32
Blood Mover
  Crampbark and Ginger Fomentation...............33
  Arnica Ointment...35
Carminative
  Chinese Five Spice Blend..............................36
  Digestive Blend...37
  Explore Carminative Herbs...........................39
  Kitchari...40
  Les Herbes de Provence................................43
  Parsley Pesto..44
Relaxing Nervine
  Comparing Basils..45
  Nutmeg Milk..46
Sialagogue
  Mouthwash..47
Stimulating Diaphoretic
  Cayenne Tea..48
  Tom Kha...49

Stimulating Diuretic
  Diuretic Tea...52
  Juniper with Caramelized Apples and Onions.....53
Stimulating Expectorant
  Elecampane Honey......................................54
  Fire Cider by Erin McIntosh..........................55
  Homemade Mustard....................................57

Salty...59
Introduction to Salty
  With and Without Salt.................................60
Nourishing Herbs
  Apple Cider Vinegar Infused with Chickweed....61
  De la Forêt Salad Dressing............................62
  Kale Chips...63
  Oatstraw Tea...64
  Stinging Nettle Eggplant Parmesan.................65
  Violet infused oil...67
Salt
  Artisanal Salts..68
  Bath Salt Blend..70
  Celery Salt..71
  Chamomile Popsicles...................................72
  Saline rinse for eyes and nose.......................74
  Salt Scrub...75
  Simple Electrolyte Blend..............................76
Seaweed
  Salmon and Seaweed Soup...........................77
  Seaweed Bath..78
  Seaweed Cookies.......................................79
  Seaweed Salt Scrub....................................80
  Sea Zest Seasoning.....................................81

Sour..83
Introduction to Sour
  Astringency Scale.......................................84
  Lemon Water..85
  Sour or Bitter?...86
Astringent
  Bay Rum Aftershave...................................87
  Facial Clay Mask..88
  Facial Toner..89
  Leaky Gut Tea...90
  Mouth Pack..91

Table of Contents

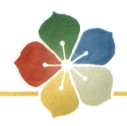

Rose Petal Vinegar..................................92
Simple Deodorant..................................94
Sitz Bath..................................95
Uterine Tonic Tea..................................96
UTI Formula..................................97
Varicose Vein Cream..................................98
Berries
Hawthorne Cordial..................................99
Limoncello..................................100
Pomegranate Molasses..................................101
Rosehip and Cranberry Compote..................102
Rosehip Preserves..................................103
Rosehip Vinegar..................................104
Sopa de Lima..................................105
Spicy Lemonade..................................107
Strawberry Rhubarb Compote..................108
Fermented
Beet Kvass..................................109
Fermented Veggies..................................110
Miso Soup..................................112
Yogurt..................................113

Bitter 115
Introduction to Sour
Bitterness Scale..................................116
Alterative & Lymphagogue
Alterative Blend..................................117
Marinated Burdock Root..................................118
Rich Roasted Reishi Tea..................................119
Dandelion Tea..................................120
Balances Blood Sugar
Bitter Melon Juice..................................121
Spiced Coffee..................................122
Laxative
Rooty Laxative..................................123
Triphala..................................124
Nervine
Herbal Dark Chocolate Truffles..................125
Chocolate Mousse Cake..................................127
Relaxing Nervines..................................128
Skullcap Tea..................................129
Sleep Blend..................................130

Relaxing Diaphoretic
Boneset Tea..................................131
Elderflower Tea..................................132
Stimulates Digestion
Creamy Greens Soup..................................133
Dandelion Pesto..................................134
Make your own bitters..................................135
Roasted Radicchio..................................137
Vermicide
Parasite Formula..................................138

Sweet 139
Introduction to Sweet
Tasting Sweet Herbs..................................140
Marshmallows..................................141
Vanilla Extract..................................143
Adaptogen
Adaptogen Bon Bons..................................145
Congee..................................147
Blood & Yin Tonic
Blood Building Syrup..................................148
Borscht..................................150
Yellow Dock Syrup..................................152
Demulcent
Marshmallow Infusion..................................153
Sore Throat Pastilles..................................154
Immunomodulator
Nourishing Bone Broth..................................157
Shitake Shallot Butter..................................158
Vulnerary
Comfrey Poultice..................................159
Plantain Salve..................................160

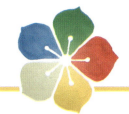

Why is the taste of herbs important?

The taste of herbs is a facet of herbalism that has intrigued me for several years. I began teaching about the Taste of Herbs three years ago with presentations alongside Michael Tierra, and I've taught an introductory course at herbal conferences across North America.

After several years of exploring the taste of herbs, I am still fascinated with sensorial exploration! I've even created an entire course exploring these concepts in depth.

Exploring herbs through the sense of taste is a traditional tool that has been used for as long as we can imagine. Before microscopes, petri dishes, and isolated chemical constituents, taste was a practical tool to give someone insight into how to use an herb.

This practice is still very much alive in traditional methods of herbalism. If you were to study herbs from an Ayurvedic or Traditional Chinese Medicine perspective, you would find that taste is an important part of studying herbs and their methods of use.

In Traditional Chinese Medicine there are five tastes.

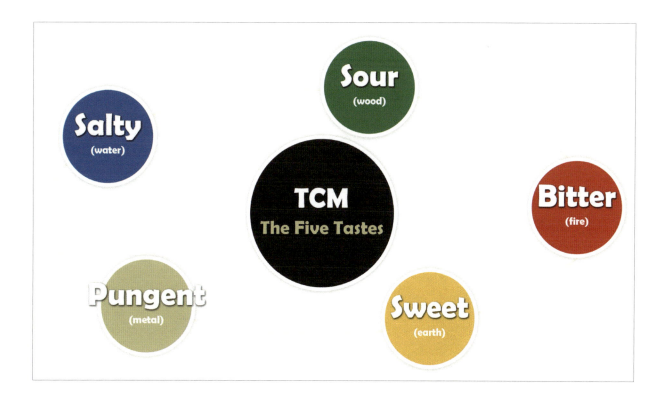

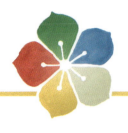

In Ayurveda there is a sixth taste, astringent. (In Traditional Chinese Medicine astringent is considered to be a part of the sour taste.)

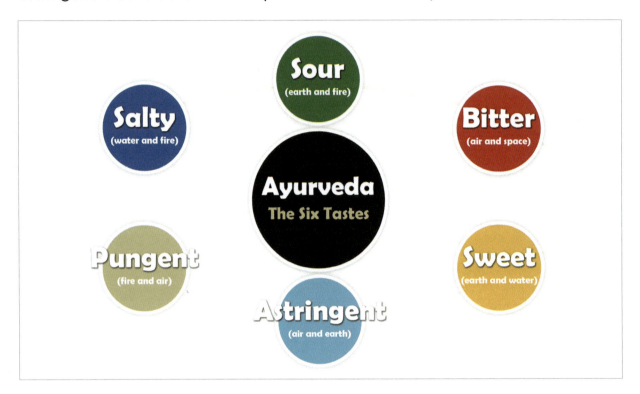

For me, studying the taste of herbs is two-fold. On the one hand it is a theory that has been passed down through many generations, and it is something that can be memorized to gain a deeper understanding of herbs and how they work.

But taste isn't something that should be learned from book study alone! Our own subjective experience of taste is just as important to explore. As Paul Bergner recommends: "To be a master herbalist in thirty years or more, taste an herb every day."

> To me, any herbalist who doesn't know the taste of an herb but attempts to use it can be compared to a painter who doesn't know the colors of the rainbow, or a musician who doesn't know the scales.
>
> Alan Keith Tillotson
> Herbalist

Here are my six top reasons why herbalists should study the Taste of Herbs!

1. Tasting herbs is about connection

Taste can give us a strong visceral connection with plants that goes beyond memorizing what books say or even what our teachers say.

Our senses - taste, touch, smell, hearing, and sight - are powerful ways in which we make sense of our world. They help us to take in information, record that information and learn.

Ever have a sense of smell immediately evoke strong memories?

Ever hear a song that instantly brings you back to a particular time in your life?

How about the taste of comfort food? A favorite family recipe?

These experiences of the senses strongly transport us to another place and time.

They present another way of knowing that strongly activates the mind. We can easily forget something we read in a book one time, but once you really connect with a plant through the sense of taste you'll never forget it.

2. The Taste of Herbs is key to understanding Herbal Energetics

In my opinion, one of the reasons herbalism is such a powerful form of medicine is that it matches herbs to people instead of diseases. As herbalists we don't diagnose eczema, fibromyalgia, or heartburn and then give herbs to match those diseases. That is more the realm of western medicine.

Instead, we seek to understand the person and their underlying imbalances and skillfully match herbs, diet, and lifestyle suggestions to help them create health from the inside out.

When using herbs in this way, they go beyond being "herbs for eczema" and become a powerful tool to help someone discover and resolve the root cause of their health problems.

Does the person have too much heat? Cold? Is there too much dryness or moisture?

Once we understand the person, we can then match herbs to the person.

Warming herbs can be given to help someone who has too much coldness. Cooling herbs can be given for someone with too much heat.

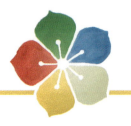

How do we know if an herb is warming or cooling?

By taste and taste sensations.

I know you already know this!

On a hot summer's day do you reach for a steaming hot bowl of chili? Or watermelon?

On a brisk fall day do you want an iced smoothie or a warm drink?

The taste of herbs is like an herbal decoder ring for understanding herbal energetics. With this knowledge you can be more confident and effective when choosing herbal remedies.

3. How potent an herb is

I often hear people ask about the potency of an herb. The classic example is someone finding a long-lost jar of herbs on their back shelf and wanting to know whether it's still good.

Since there isn't really a broadly accepted "due date" on herbs, the best way to tell is by using our senses. If you know how the herb tastes when it's vibrant and potent herbal medicine, then you can do a taste comparison to tell if you can use your forgotten herb with confidence or if it's too far past its prime.

You can also use the sense of taste to determine if the herbs you harvested from your garden are more or less potent than the herbs you bought online or the herbs you wildcrafted.

I love being able to taste an herb or an herbal preparation and know by taste alone whether or not it is going to be powerful medicine.

4. If it's the right herb

Most of the time we confidently know which herb we have. Perhaps we harvested it ourselves using our plant ID skills, or it came fully labeled from a reputable company. Sometimes we can simply use our eyes to know that yes, this is really chamomile.

But this isn't always the case. The majority of herbal safety problems comes from adulterated herbs. This is where someone has substituted a more readily

available herb that looks similar to the one desired. Skullcap being adulterated with germander is a key example.

Powdered herbs can be difficult to recognize by sight alone. Knowing the taste of an herb can help you to really know that the powdered herbs you get are the ones you ordered.

Another way you can use taste to know if it is the right herb is fairly obscure. I am sure this would never apply to anyone reading this. But let's just say that perhaps someone, at sometime, forgot to label one of their herbs or herbal preparations. If they intimately know the taste of herbs then they'll be able to tell if that green jar of tincture is California Poppy or Skullcap. (Note: this is for example purposes only and has, of course, never happened to me.)

5. Commonalities between species

Another frequent question people have is whether they can use a plant with the same genus, but different species, in a similar way.

What about plantains? Can *Plantago lanceolata* be used similarly to *Plantago major*?

Can *Rosa rugosa* be used like *Rosa nootka*?

Can common mallow (*Malva neglecta*) be used like marshmallow (*Althaea officinalis*)?

One way to tell the difference is by taste!

Do they taste the same? Do they feel the same in your body?

6. Differences between species or even plant parts

Just as the taste of an herb can tell us if two similar herbs can be used in the same way, the taste of herbs can tell us if they are different.

Is *Monarda dydima* similar to *Monarda fistulosa*? Or is Holy Basil similar to culinary basil? The answer to this is fairly obvious once you know their taste.

The taste of herbs can also gives us insight into whether different parts of a plant can be used in similar ways. For example, can elecampane flowers be used like elecampane root? What's the difference between valerian flowers and valerian root?

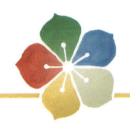

Summary

Understanding how the taste of herbs can be used in theory and in practice provides herbalists with a practical tool that they can use every day. Not only can it increase your confidence and effectiveness when choosing herbal remedies, it can also bring herbs to life through a sensorial and visceral connection to the plants.

> "As in ancient times, herbalists would do well to continue to rely upon their trained senses and experience to properly assess the therapeutic nature of plants, and among the different faculties there is perhaps no equal to the perception of taste.
>
> Used by every system of traditional medicine, taste figures prominently in the practice of herbal medicine, providing immediate insight into the properties and uses of medicinal plants."
>
> Todd Caldecott
> Herbalist

The 5 Tastes

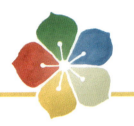

Tips for tasting herbs...

1. Consciously use your sense of taste each day. Think of it as a muscle you want to strengthen.

2. When tasting, set aside some quiet space where you can reflect. (If that's not possible for you, taste anyway!)

3. Keep of journal of your tastes. Write down what you are tasting—a quick note, obsevation, or question on how you are feeling that day.

4. Smell the herb you are tasting.

5. Feel how it tastes on your tongue. Do you notice one predominate taste? Secondary tastes.

6. Feel where it goes in your body. Do you notice yourself taking a deeper breath? Do you feel the digestive process begin? (More salivation, tummy rumbling?) There are no wrong answers, just notice what you feel.

7. Do you have a sense of whether this herb is warming or cooling? Drying or moistening?

8. Taste herbs in a variety of different preparations.
    - fresh
    - dried
    - tea (strong tea/weak tea)
    - roasted
    - in food
    - tinctures
    - vinegar extracts
    - honey extracts
    - syrup
    - and on and on and on

9. Research what others say about the taste of this herb. Don't disqualify your own observation if it differs from a book. Remember it's all subjective and is simply information in the exploration process.

PUNGENT

Ayurveda Elements

Fire and Wind
hot, dry and light

TCM Organs

Lungs and Large Intestine
yang

Chemical constituents

essential oils, resins

How we use the pungent taste

Pungent foods are stimulating, warming, and drying. They are dispersing and can relieve stagnant digestion (gas, bloating) and increase metabolism. They are often used for fevers (with coldness) and to stimulate expectoration.

Examples

Pungent tastes are found in many culinary spices such as pepper, ginger, basil, rosemary, garlic, clove, and cayenne.

Contraindications

Heat, dryness, burning sensations.

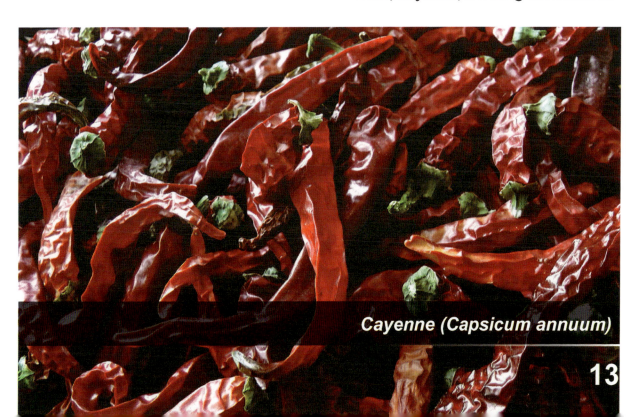

Cayenne (Capsicum annuum)

EXERCISE, PUNGENT

Exercise 1: Discovering Diffusive Herbs

Understanding the diffusive sensation of pungent tastes is crucial.

I recommend that you taste prickly ash tincture to experience what that intense quality is. If you don't have access to prickly ash consider tasting other diffusive herbs.

Extra credit

Choose 3-5 diffusive herbs and spend time tasting each of them.

Next, rate these herbs on a scale. Which were the most diffusive to you? The least? How else did they differ? Were some hotter than others? Did you notice one having a particular organ affinity?

List of diffusive herbs

- Sage (*Salvia officinalis*)
- Thyme (*Thymus vulgaris*)
- Prickly Ash (*Xanthoxylum americanum*)
- Ginger (*Zingiber officinalis*)
- Most aromatic mints
- Dill (*Anethum graveolens*)
- Fennel (*Foeniculum vulgare*)
- Burdock seeds (*Arctium lappa*)
- Cinnamon (*Cinnamomum zeylanicum*)
- Turmeric (*Curcuma longa*)
   - Cayenne (*Capsicum annuum*)

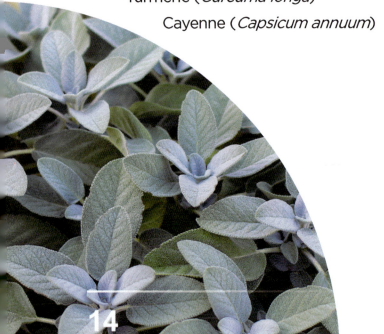

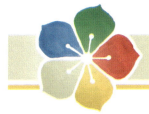

EXERCISE, PUNGENT

Exercise 2: Fresh Ginger vs. Dried Ginger

I am frequently asked what's the difference between using fresh ginger and dried ginger? In this exercise you'll get to find out using your own sense of taste and experience!

HERE'S WHAT YOU'LL NEED...

- 1 tablespoon of freshly minced fresh ginger
- 2 teaspoons of dried ginger
- 16 ounces of water (just-boiled)
- two identical mugs or cups

In this exercise, you are going to brew two identical cups of tea. On the bottom of each cup, use masking tape to label whether you are putting in dried or fresh ginger.

In one cup, place the teaspoon of freshly minced ginger in the cup marked fresh.

In the other cup, place 1/2 teaspoon of cut and dried ginger in the cup marked dried.

Pour 8 ounces of just-boiled water into each cup. Cover and let them steep for 10 minutes.

Strain both cups. Mix them around so that you no longer know which one is fresh and which one is dried.

Choose one cup and sip it. Experience the sensations without judgment, just awareness.

Try the other cup. Experience the sensations with awareness.

Go back and forth between the two, taking a break as needed so that your palate is still discerning.

What do you notice about the differences?

Make a guess as to which is fresh and which is dried. Were you right?

Why do you think I suggested using half as much dried ginger to the fresh ginger?

What are the different sensations you felt?

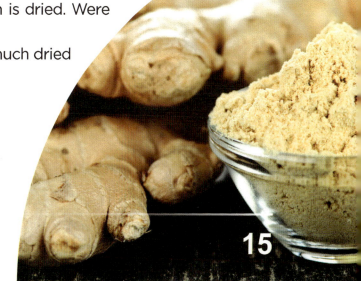

EXERCISE, PUNGENT

Exercise 3: Tasting Ginger

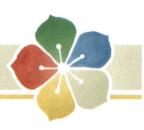

This exercise is a further exploration of the diffusive sensation and is really about further training your herbalist senses. It may seem overly simple, but I promise you I've had some of my biggest "Ahas" with this practice.

WHAT YOU'LL NEED...

- 4 teaspoons dried ginger
- 8 ounces of just-boiled water
- mug

Place the ginger in the cup. Pour in the water. Cover and let it steep for 10 minutes. Strain.

Sit in a quiet space where you can focus on your experience.

Sip the tea gingerly (pun intended). What do you notice? Do you feel the heat of the tea sink to your belly? What happens after that?

Notice your experience.

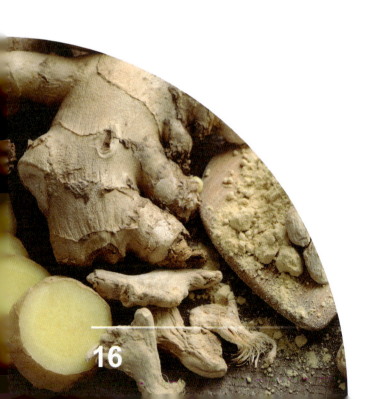

EXERCISE, PUNGENT

Exercise 4: Tincture vs. Tea

Ever wonder if taking a tincture is the same as taking a tea? That is a great question with no easy answer. It really depends on the person, the herb, the situation, etc. In this exercise we'll explore the variety of tastes within different ginger preparations.

This practice can easily be expanded to other herbs.

WHAT YOU'LL NEED...

- ginger tincture
- 60 drops of ginger tincture squirted into 8 ounces of hot water
- warm ginger tea (prepared with 2 teaspoons of fresh or dried ginger and 8 ounces of water)
- cool ginger tea (prepared with 2 teaspoons of fresh or dried ginger and 8 ounces of water)

With all four preparations in front of you, take time to taste each of them.

What do you notice? Do they taste differently? What are the different sensations you experience?

Record your experiences and thoughts about this exercise. Remember, there are no wrong answers just awareness!

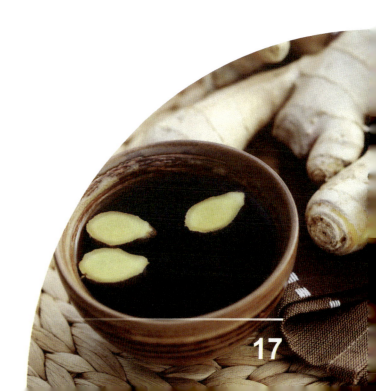

EXERCISE, ANODYNE

Cayenne Salve

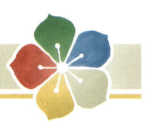

This super simple salve can be made up very quickly and bring big-time pain relief. The heating quality of cayenne moves blood and stagnancy (which can cause pain) and it also blocks Substance P, the neuropeptide that can relay the pain signal.

WHAT YOU'LL NEED...

- 1/2 cup olive oil
- two heaping teaspoons of cayenne powder (or 15 grams)
- 1/2 ounce of beeswax
- double boiler
- cheesecloth

Begin by infusing the cayenne into the olive oil over a double boiler. Heat the oil and cayenne until it's warm. Turn off the heat and let it sit (warmly) for about 20 minutes, then turn the heat on again. Do this for at least 1 hour to a couple of hours. You could do it for 24 hours if desired.

Once the cayenne and olive oil have been infused, strain off the powder through a cheesecloth. Reserve the infused oil.

Heat the beeswax until it's melted. Stir in the infused oil until the beeswax and oil have been thoroughly melted together and combined.

Immediately pour this mixture into jars or tins (it makes roughly 4 ounces). Let it cool and then label it.

USING YOUR CAYENNE SALVE

This cayenne salve can be used on aches and pains, from sore muscles and joints to bruises, and even nerve pain. It's best for closed wounds and may sting a bit on open wounds. Even on closed skin you may feel a bit of burning or heat in the area where it is used. It should be applied externally only and used within 6 months for the best results.

If using it for arthritic pain, it may take up to a week or two to see results. Use it daily to decrease chronic pain.

Caution: When cayenne comes in contact with your mucosal membranes or eyes it will burn! Be sure to wash your hands thoroughly after touching cayenne or use gloves to apply the salve to the desired area. If you are using the cayenne salve on your hands, consider applying it at night and then sleeping with gloves on.

Some people with thin or sensitive skin may find that cayenne salve causes blistering. If this happens, stop use until it heals, then resume using a smaller amount, or remake the salve using less cayenne.

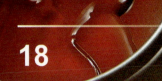

EXERCISE, ANODYNE

Basic Camphor and Menthol Pain Salve

Camphor and menthol are fantastic for relieving acute pain. This recipe uses them in an oil base that is hardened into a salve.

I like to use herb-infused oils for this, cottonwood being one of my favorites. Your own favorite herbal pain relievers can be used as well.

WHAT YOU'LL NEED...

- 1 cup oil (optional herb-infused oil)
- 1 ounce beeswax
- 20 grams coconut oil
- 1/2 tablespoon of menthol crystals
- 1/2 tablespoon of camphor crystals

Heat the beeswax and coconut oil in a double boiler or on really low heat.

Once it's melted, remove from heat and add the 1/2 tablespoon camphor and 1/2 tablespoon menthol. Stir until dissolved. (I like to use a popsicle stick that I then throw away.)

Add the oil. If necessary add a bit more heat until everything is melted.

Pour into jars or tins and label for external use.

To use: rub it into the affected area. Then, cover that area with something you don't mind getting oily such as old clothing or a scarf.

Wash your hands after use to avoid accidentally getting it into your eyes or sensitive mucous membranes.

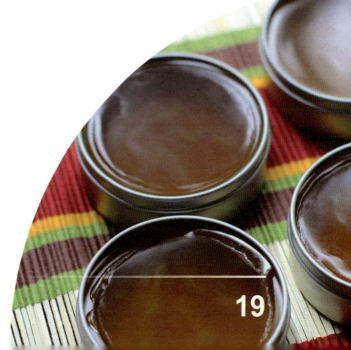

EXERCISE, ANTIMICROBIAL

Bee Balm Oxymel

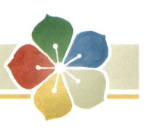

Bee balm has many names: Sweet leaf, wild bergamot, horsemint, wild oregano, and oswego tea being a few examples, but all refer to the *Monarda genus*.

Endemic to North America and easily grown in the garden, this is one of our very own native culinary spices. Mostly spicy with a hint of sweetness, bee balm can be added to all sorts of dishes to give it a special local flavoring.

But don't let the words "culinary spice" fool you. This is one of our most potent herbal remedies for all sorts of infections. It can be used for bladder infections, yeast infections, topical fungal infections, it's used in steam for congested sinuses, it can be used as a mouthwash for gum infections, and used for a variety of symptomatic complaints of the cold and flu.

As an antimicrobial herb, it works wonderfully as a tea or infused honey on a sore and inflamed throat.

As a diaphoretic herb, it can support the fever process by increasing internal warmth while someone feels cold and is shivering. Bee balm is a diffusive herb. It brings heat from the core of the body to the periphery. If that sounds abstract to you, try drinking a cup of hot bee balm tea. You can literally feel the heat rise from the core of your body up to the skin and then dissipate. That's diffusive!

Do you use oil of oregano for infections? Before you reach for that expensive bottle, think of bee balm!

> "Oil of Oregano is currently a popular item in alternative medicine for combating candida and various infections, but what most people do not know is that the active constituent of Oil of Oregano is present in large amounts in our own Monarda. For anything you might use Oil of Oregano for, you can substitute the prolific (and cheap) Monarda."
>
> Kiva Rose
> Oxymels

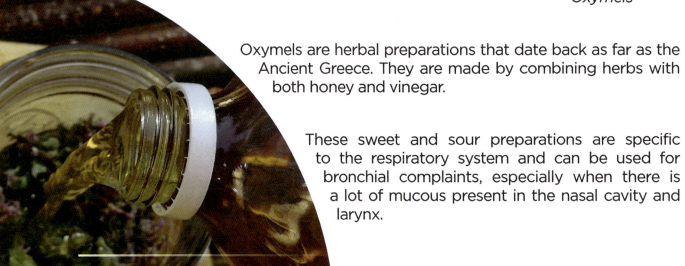

Oxymels are herbal preparations that date back as far as the Ancient Greece. They are made by combining herbs with both honey and vinegar.

These sweet and sour preparations are specific to the respiratory system and can be used for bronchial complaints, especially when there is a lot of mucous present in the nasal cavity and larynx.

I learned from herbalist Paul Bergner that William Cook, a Physiomedicalist of the 1800s, preferred vinegar as a menstruum for issues of the respiratory system. He felt that it concentrated the herb's actions to the respiratory system.

Honey, in itself, offers us a wide range of benefits for coughs and sore throats. It's antimicrobial, inhibiting the growth of pathogens, as well as slightly expectorant. As most of us know, a spoonful of honey can soothe a sore throat.

WHAT YOU'LL NEED...

- Fresh or dried bee balm (bee balm is difficult to find in commerce; thyme, oregano or rosemary can be substituted in this recipe)
- organic apple cider vinegar
- local raw honey

You can use fresh herbs or dried herbs for this recipe. I harvested the leaves and flowers of my bee balm and then let it wilt for a couple of days.

Once it had lost some of its water content (wilted), I chopped it up and filled a jar 3/4 of the way full.

If you are using completely fresh herbs, you may want to fill the entire jar with them. If you are using dried herbs, I would start with filling it half full.

Now it's time to add the honey and vinegar. There is some room to play here. I prefer my mixture to be less sweet, so I added about 1/3 of the jar full of honey and the rest full of vinegar.

You can make this, however, try half honey and half vinegar for more experimentation. Or even more honey than vinegar. Try making several batches in smaller jars to see what you like best.

Once you've got the honey and vinegar added, stir it well.

Use a plastic lid to cover the oxymel or use a metal lid, but put wax paper in between the metal and the liquid. Vinegar will corrode metal and make your oxymel unusable.

I continue to stir mine for several days to make sure it's all mixed together. After a bit of time, the honey and vinegar will mix together well forming a consistent liquid.

Let this sit for at least two weeks, preferably for a month. Shake or stir it often during this time.

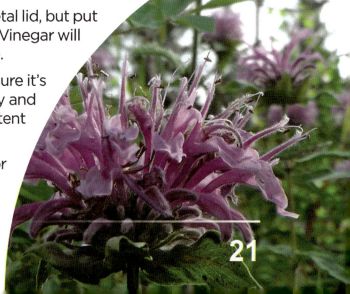

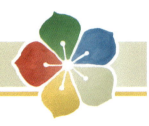

Once it's infused for long enough (or you get sick and need to use it), you can strain off the herbal material, OR you can leave it in. If you are using fresh herbs, it can be pleasant to leave them in. But sometimes dried herbs are better strained out.

This mixture can be used by the spoonful as needed for thick congested coughs, sore throats, and general support during a cold or flu.

If you used fresh herbs, store this mixture in the fridge or a cool place. It should last for a year, possibly longer.

And if you are fortunate to not fall ill this year, try it as a salad dressing mix or as part of a marinade on meats or vegetables.

Bee balm is safe for most people to use, but if you have special health conditions, you may want to check with an herbalist before using it. It shouldn't be used in large quantities.

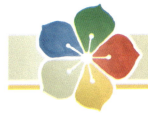

EXERCISE, ANTIMICROBIAL

Cold Sore Lip Balm

I learned this fabulous recipe from herbalist and aromatherapist Jade Shutes from the East West School of Aromatherapy. Both the essential oils in this recipe are scientifically proven to be effective against the herpes virus, plus the recipe nourishes the lips

When buying lemon balm essential oil, it's very important to get it from a reputable source. Lemon balm essential oil is a bit expensive. If you find it for cheap then it is probably either a synthetic oil or has been adulterated with some other essential oil.

WHAT YOU'LL NEED...

- 20 grams of beeswax
- 40 grams of jojoba or sesame oil (or 10 grams tamanu oil and 30 grams sesame oil)
- 25 grams of shea butter or coconut oil
- 15 grams of cocoa butter
- 25 drops Melissa (*Melissa officinalis*) essential oil
- 10 drops *Eucalyptus globulus* essential oil

Begin by melting the beeswax on low heat or in a double boiler.

Once it is melted, stir in the oils and butter. Stir until the solid ingredients are completely melted. Remove from heat.

Add the essential oils. Stir well.

Pour into lip balm tubs or metal tins.

Makes approxitemately 10-12 tubes of lip balm. These keep for about a year, possibly longer if stored in a cool location.

EXERCISE, ANTIMICROBIAL

Vinegar Cleaner

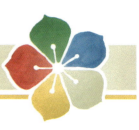

In our efforts to bring freshness into our homes, it would be silly to use harsh chemical cleaning agents. Yet this is what many people do in an attempt to create a sterile home environment. I avoid walking down the cleaning aisle at the grocery store. Otherwise, that harsh cacophony of scents assuredly reddens my eyes and gives me a headache. No thank you!

Even "natural" cleaners you buy at the grocery store can include not-so-natural chemicals and cost a pretty penny.

In this exercise we are going to make a 100% natural herbal cleaner that is super effective at cleaning counters, stove tops, and bathroom appliances. Better yet, this cleaner will undoubtedly cost you less than $5 for a year's supply!

Before we get to the recipe let's learn more about our ingredients.

Vinegar
In this recipe we'll be using distilled white vinegar. You can buy this at grocery stores, and it's fairly cheap at $2-4 a gallon. Vinegar could be the only cleaner you'll ever need. It can clean practically everything, from the toilet to the windows (just switch out rags in between). I don't get caught up worrying about germs but, if that is a concern for you, white vinegar is a natural disinfectant.

Thyme
Many of us think of thyme as simply a culinary herb, but thyme has a well-deserved place in our medicine cabinet as well. Thyme tea is fabulous for lung congestion and coughs. I've used it for productive coughs (to loosen and expel mucous) as well as for dry spasmodic coughs (to lessen the cough). Antimicrobial in nature, it has been used for centuries to clean wounds and kill parasitic fungi on the skin. These antimicrobial properties make it great for cleaning your house as well.

Lavender
Its lovely scent is sweet enough for linen sachets and calming enough to relieve stress. I'll admit that the soothing smell of lavender makes cleaning all the happier. The word lavender comes from the Latin word lavare which means "to wash". It has been used for bathing for eons. It's antimicrobial, making it another wonderful addition to our cleaning crew.

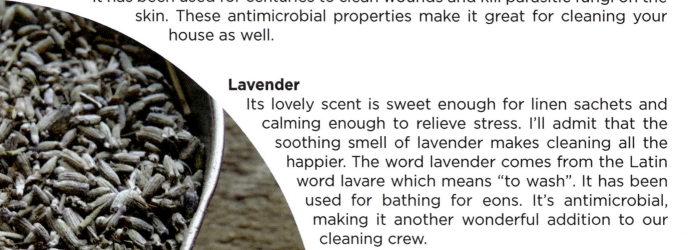

WHAT YOU'LL NEED...

- 1 quart of vinegar
- 1 cup of dried thyme leaves and flowers
- 1 cup of dried lavender flowers
- quart jar

Place the dried herbs in a quart jar.

Fill the jar with vinegar. Cover with a plastic lid (not metal).

Let this sit for 24 hours. The next day, the vinegar should be a lovely red color, which comes from the thyme.

Strain out the vinegar well, and place it in a spray bottle.

Voila! You have your own super cheap, super effective herbal vinegar cleaner.

We use this exclusively in our house to clean the stove, countertops, kitchen sink, toilet, windows, etc. It cuts through grease and leaves a pleasant scent. If desired, you could even add some essential oils to the vinegar as well.

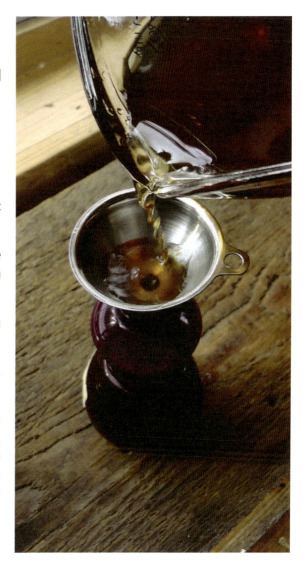

EXERCISE, ANTISPASMODIC

Antispasmodic liniment

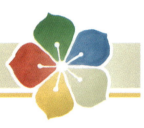

Got muscle tension? Crick in your neck? Tight shoulders? Leg cramp? This is a wonderful liniment that helps relax spasmodic muscles. It gently relieves pain from muscle tension by combining antispasmodic herbs with warming blood herbs.

Liniments are alcohol extracts that are for external use only. Sometimes people use isopropyl alcohol in these solutions, but I prefer to use regular alcohol tinctures.

This recipe makes four ounces of liniment.

WHAT YOU'LL NEED...

- 1 ounce of Kava tincture
- 1 ounce of Jamaican Dogwood tincture
- 1 ounce of Cramp bark tincture
- 1 ounce of Ginger tincture
- 5 drops of Eucalyptus essential oil
- 10 drops of Peppermint Essential oil

Combine all the ingredients together.

Label for external use only.

To use this liniment spray it over the effected area and gently rub it in.

Repeat as needed.

A hot water bottle may also be applied to the area for added relief.

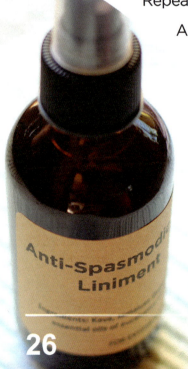

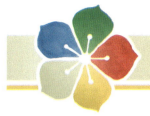

EXERCISE, ANTISPASMODIC

Cramp bark Chai

If you know me at all, you'll know how much I love chai teas. During the winter months we practically have chai brewing on the wood stove. I love how versatile chai teas can be. They can be used simply as a warming digestive aid that tastes great, or they can be used to mask the unpleasant flavors of other herbs.

This cramp bark chai is a nice blend for people with muscle tension. I especially use it for people with menstrual cramps. The chai spices and the cramp bark all help relieve the tension and pain associated with menstrual cramps.

WHAT YOU'LL NEED...

- 1 tablespoon of cramp bark
- 2 tablespoons of ginger root
- 2 tablespoons of dried orange peel
- 1 tablespoon of cinnamon chips
- 1 teaspoon of peppercorns
- 1/2 teaspoon of hulled cardamom or two crushed cardamom pods
- 1/4 teaspoon of cloves (about 3-5 cloves)
- 1 & 1/2 quarts of water
- optional: milk and honey

Place all the ingredients in a pan. Bring to a boil, then lower the heat.

Cover and simmer for one hour. Strain. Add the milk and honey, if desired.

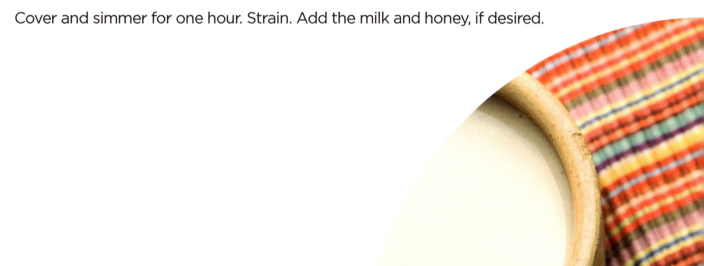

EXERCISE, ANXIOLYTIC

Kava Hot Cocoa

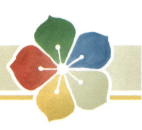

Kava *(Piper methysticum)* comes to us from the Pacific Islands. It has a long traditional and ceremonial use dating back thousands of years.

The root of the kava plant is used as a beverage and it was traditionally prepared by mastication or chewing of the root. When Europeans made contact with the Pacific Islanders they discouraged this practice. Now, we know that mastication makes a potent brew!

Kava can be a little tricky to work with. It doesn't like heat, and the alcohol percentage in a tincture is very specific. The recipe below calls for kneading the powdered root in cold water.

Kava is a wonderful relaxing nervine. It can relax muscles and give a sense of calm. A friend recently described drinking kava to getting a luxurious massage. That's a pretty good description!

Kava can also be used for acute pain due to spasms such as kidney stones or menstrual cramping.

Chocolate is a good source of magnesium. Magnesium can stop muscle spasms and also promotes a sense of calm. The two go together quite well!

If you've never had kava before, you'll quickly notice a very distinct acrid taste and numbing sensation on your tongue. If the kava doesn't produce this effect, it probably wasn't prepared right.

Recently, kava made the sensational news headlines as being a dangerous herb. It's true that kava contains some potent alkaloids. However, in all cases where injury was established, it was from extracts that had potentiated certain constituents of the kava root (kavalactones). There have been no injuries associated with appropriate use of the whole plant. However, it is contraindicated in pregnancy, breastfeeding, and those with liver disease. If you visit Jim Mcdonald's incredible article index and search for "kava", you'll see many articles on the safety of kava. *http://www.herbcraft.org/articleindex.html*

Please do not buy wild harvested kava. Get it from a sustainable cultivated source. You can find fresh kava here: *http://www.nukahivatrading.com/*

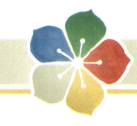

WHAT YOU'LL NEED...

- 1/2 cup powdered Kava root
- 1/2 cup fair trade cocoa powder
- 6 cups water
- 1 tablespoon vanilla
- 1 teaspoon cinnamon
- Honey and cream to taste

Step One: Make the Kava

Place 1/2 cup of kava powder into a muslin bag.

Place the bag in a large bowl along with 4 cups of water (lukewarm).

Knead the bag for an extended period of time. How long? 20 minutes should do, however, waiting longer could be better.

Once you feel that you are done kneading, you can start making the cocoa. The kava mixture should look cloudy. Note: you are now done using the muslin bag and it can be repurposed.

Step Two: Make the cocoa

Combine the cocoa, cinnamon and water into a small saucepan and heat on medium high, stirring constantly. Once the cocoa has dissolved and while the temperature is fairly warm, remove from heat.

Step Three: Combining the two

I like to mix equal parts of cocoa to cloud the kava mixture, but you can mix it up anyway you like. I add cream and honey to taste.

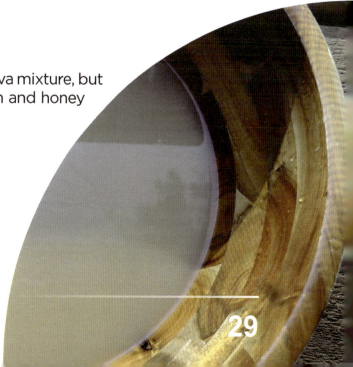

EXERCISE, APHRODISIAC

Cardamom and Chia Seed Pudding

If you have never had chia seed pudding, you are in for a treat! Chia seeds are nutritious seeds that soak up the liquid around them to form a tapioca-like pudding. This recipe uses one of my favorite aphrodisiac herbs, cardamom, to make a romantic dessert with chia seeds.

This recipe takes only minutes to put together, but then it needs several hours or overnight for it to turn into a pudding.

WHAT YOU'LL NEED...

- 1/3 cup chia seeds
- one 13.5 ounce can of coconut milk
- 13.5 ounces of water
- 1-2 tablespoons cardamom powder
- honey to taste

In a medium sized bowl, stir together the water and coconut milk until it is an even consistency.

Add the chia seeds and mix well. Let stand for one hour in the fridge, then stir again, breaking up any clusters of chia seeds if necessary. Store for a couple more hours, or overnight, in the fridge before serving.

Add the cardamom powder and honey to taste. Mix well.

Serve chilled. Keeps in the fridge for several days.

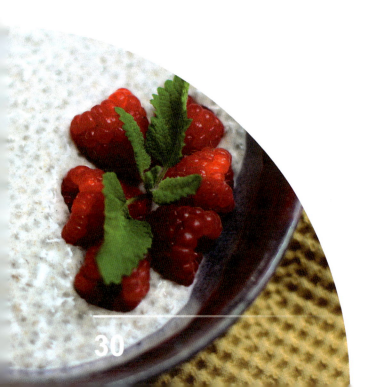

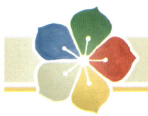

EXERCISE, APHRODISIAC

Damiana Tea

Damiana is an infamous plant that has been used for centuries by the Mayans and Aztecs. It is considered to be a safe herb, but because it has been used by some as an alternative to marijuana, it has been banned outright in the state of Louisiana!

Damiana is best known for its aphrodisiac qualities. It is often lauded as the herbal equivalent to viagra and is commonly sold as a sexual enhancement supplement. While damiana is deserving of its aphrodisiac reputation, as herbalists we know better than to think of herbs like drugs!

Damiana is nourishing and supporting for sexual health. It is commonly taken as a tea and blends well with other nourishing and aphrodisiac herbs.

WHAT YOU'LL NEED...

- 1 tablespoon of damiana leaves
- 1 tablespoon of oats
- 1 tablespoon of rose petals
- pinch of stevia (optional)
- 8 ounces of just-boiled water.

Place the herbs in a cup. Pour in the just-boiled water.

Cover and let it steep for 10-15 minutes. Strain.

Sweeten with honey, if desired.

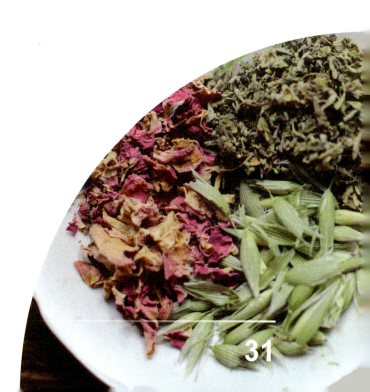

EXERCISE, APHRODISIAC

Sexy Chai Blend

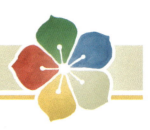

This chai blend is spicy! It warms the body and arouses the mind. This can be drunk daily, especially during the colder months of the year.

In the wintertime I cook my chai teas on the wood stove to conserve energy. Another method is to put it in the crock pot on low overnight. That way you wake up to an evocative smell throughout the house and a warm chai for breakfast.

WHAT YOU'LL NEED...

- 2 tablespoons of burdock root
- 2 tablespoons of ginger root
- 2 tablespoons of dried orange peel
- 1 tablespoon of cinnamon chips
- 1 teaspoon of peppercorns
- 1/2 teaspoon of hulled cardamom or two crushed cardamom pods
- 1/4 teaspoon of cloves (about 3-5 cloves)
- rose water to taste
- 1 & 1/2 quarts of water

Place all the ingredients in a pan. Bring to a boil, then lower heat. Cover and simmer for one hour. Strain. Add rose water, milk and honey, if desired.

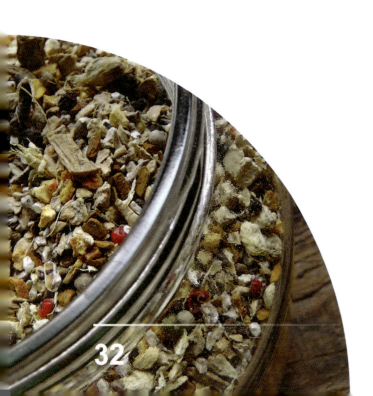

EXERCISE, BLOOD MOVING

Crampbark and Ginger Fomentation

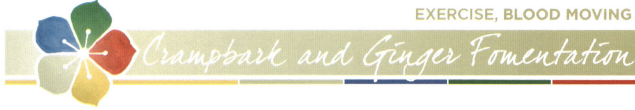

After reading this article, I bet there will be a few of you out there thinking, "Why go to all the trouble? Why not simply pop some ibuprofen?"

Most people tend to think of over-the-counter medicines as being safe. However, According to the American Gastroenterological Association (AGA), each year the side effects of NSAIDs hospitalize over 100,000 people and kill 16,500 people in the U.S. alone.

I don't know about you, but that doesn't feel very safe to me!

Cramp bark can be a reliable and safe alternative to NSAIDs. It specifically helps relax tissues and relieve tension.

In fact, cramp bark is used for the following issues: menstrual cramps, muscle cramps, early labor, miscarriage, pain, difficulty urinating, bowel cramps (IBS), diarrhea, child enuresis (bedwetting), spasmodic coughing, asthma, arthritis, muscle strain, seizures, high blood pressure, and lockjaw (interesting historic use).

I often reach for cramp bark when I've got back pain.

Have you ever "thrown out your back"?

I have, countless times.

One minute you're doing a seemingly innocent thing like picking something off the floor (or you're totally overdoing it when gardening) and bam! Something slips out of place, and the pain increases steadily until lifting your pinky finger creates excruciating pain.

After a while, the muscles around the area seize up, which immobilizes you even more.

This forced immobility is not necessarily a bad thing! Those seized muscles are protecting this vulnerable area. The holistic approach here is rest! Popping some pills or herbs and then heading back out to the garden is not a good idea, and it can injure you further.

I often use cramp bark as a fomentation over cramped muscles when I've thrown out my back.

My back and I rest staying mostly immobilized. The cramp bark fomentation significantly decreases the discomfort, but I am also not going to push myself too much and increase the risk of further injury.

Fomen-what?

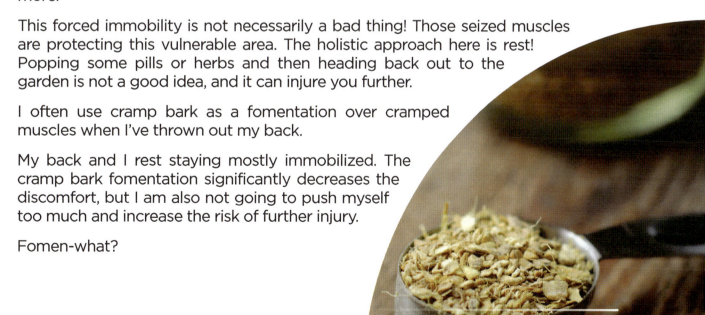

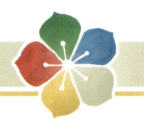

A fomentation is basically a strained herbal decoction that is then applied to the area using a cloth.

This fomentation works well for major pain, but can help with more common muscle spasms as well. For example, it can be used when you sleep wrong and have a "crick" in your neck (usually a muscle spasm). Or it can be used over the abdomen for menstrual cramps.

Besides, I add cramp bark to ginger and cayenne to this mix, also. Both of these herbs stimulate circulation (blood moving) and reduce inflammation. This combination has helped me through many painful situations!

WHAT YOU'LL NEED...

- 1/4 cup dried ginger
- 1/4 cup cramp bark
- 1 tablespoon of cayenne powder

Simmer the herbs in water for at least twenty minutes.

Strain. Let cool until you can touch it comfortably, but it's still warm.

Soak a washcloth in the mixture.

Wring out the cloth so that it is no longer dripping.

Cover the affected area with the cloth.

Place a hot water bottle over the cloth.

Cover with a towel. Let this sit for at least 20 minutes.

Sometimes I leave mine on for an hour. It feels so good!

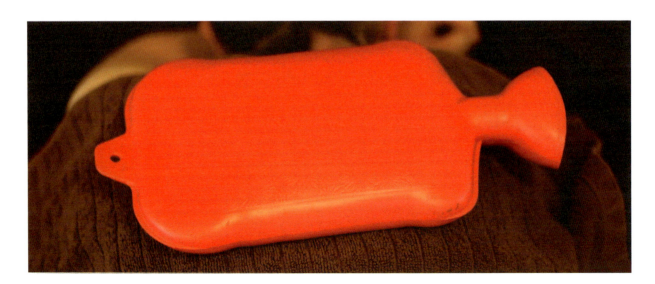

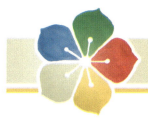

EXERCISE, BLOOD MOVING
Arnica Ointment

This is a non-greasy pain ointment that is wonderful for bruises, injuries, aches, and pains. It works best on closed-wound injuries and can be applied multiple times per day.

This recipe is based on Rosemary Gladstar's Perfect Cream recipe, but uses a tincture or liniment in place of the "waters" portion. I've seen this recipe work like magic to erase intense bruises and to alleviate aches and pains.

While you can commonly buy arnica-infused oil, arnica liniment can be harder to come by in commerce. Make your own or substitute another pain-relieving tincture such as St. John's Wort (great for nerve pain) or willow.

WHAT YOU'LL NEED...

- *Butter and wax*
    - 20 grams beeswax
    - 25 grams coconut oil
    - 20 grams shea butter
- *Oils*
    - 3/4 cup arnica-infused oil (I like using grapefruit or jojoba oils for a less greasy feel than olive oil.) Another option is to use 1/2 cup arnica-infused oil and 1/4 cup cottonwood bud infused oil.
- *"Waters"*
    - 2/3 cup arnica tincture
    - 20-40 drops of lavender essential oil

Begin by melting the butters, oil, and wax on low. Once everything is completely melted, stir in the oil. Turn off heat and stir until everything is completely mixed together.

Pour into a blender or food processor. Let sit until it has cooled and has just barely turned to a more solid state.

Turn the blender/food processor on. Slowly trickle in the arnica tincture and essential oil. It will slowly turn from a translucent mixture to a solid cream. Voila!

Store this in a glass container. This recipe makes about 12 ounces, and it should keep for about a year. Storing in the fridge or a cool location can prolong its shelf-life.

Arnica is a low-dose botanical and should not be used internally unless someone has been thoroughly trained in how to do so. Be sure to wash all the items that came in contact with the ointment very thoroughly.

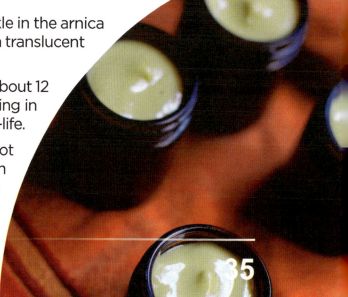

EXERCISE, CARMINATIVE

Chinese Five Spice Blend

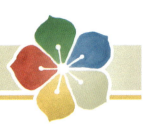

This is one example of this famous Chinese restaurant blend. Feel free to try using more or less of a spice or even add some other favorite spices.

I recommend making this in small batches so that it stays very fresh when you use it. Most powdered herbs lose their umph fairly quickly, but this should last for several months.

WHAT YOU'LL NEED...

- 2 whole star anise
- 2 teaspoons peppercorns
- 1 teaspoon cloves
- 1 teaspoon fennel seeds
- 1/2 tablespoon cinnamon chips

In a dry pan over medium heat, toast the anise, peppercorns, cloves, and fennel until fragrant. Swirl the pan gently and toss the seeds occasionally to prevent burning. This takes 2-3 minutes. Allow it to cool.

Add the spices to a spice grinder. I grind mine for about 30 seconds to get all the spices ground into a consistent soft powder.

Store this blend in an airtight spice jar and out of the light.

Try this on meats, veggies, and even popcorn.

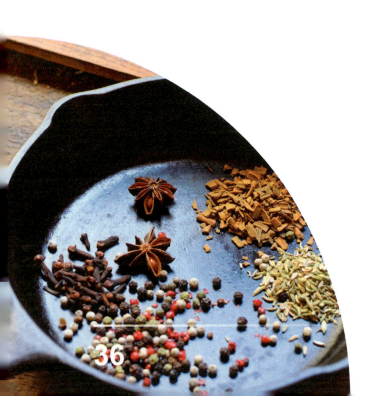

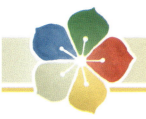

EXERCISE, CARMINATIVE

Digestive Blend

I created this tasty digestive blend with inspiration from the candied fennel jars that you often see at Indian restaurants.

Before we get to the recipe, here's some more information about the plants we'll be using.

Ginger

I probably don't have to tell many of you that ginger is one of my most favorite herbs. Spicy and diffusive herb is one of those herbs that is well suited to a myriad of woes, especially if the person has symptoms of stagnancy or coldness such as bloating, feeling colder than others in the room, and a white coating on the tongue.

Ginger is great as a digestive herb. One of its most well known uses is for nausea and for settling an upset stomach. Ginger is aromatic and diffusive, helping to nudge along stagnant digestion with symptoms of bloating, gas and bad breath. As a powerful anti-microbial herb, it can address pathogens in the digestive system as well.

One reason I end up recommending ginger to a lot of people is that it's easy to find at grocery stores, and most people enjoy the taste. For those people who aren't herbalists or consider ginger consumption as bizarre, ginger is an accessible and effective herb.

Sometimes ginger is too spicy for people with excess heat symptoms. If you avoid spicy Mexican food and Wasabi sauce, then ginger probably isn't the herb for you. For this recipe you can simply use less or omit it.

Fennel

As a medicinal herb, fennel often gets its claim to fame by helping soothe infants with colic who are distressed due to gas and other digestive discomforts. Of course, what works for our littlest ones also works quite well for us. This carminative herb works to dispel gas and promote digestion.

Fennel is a strong anti-spasmodic herb. It is often formulated with laxative herbs like rhubarb and senna because it counteracts the griping or stomach cramps often caused by these strong cathartic plants.

Like ginger, fennel is also anti-microbial. It has even been shown to be effective in drug-resistant tuberculosis.

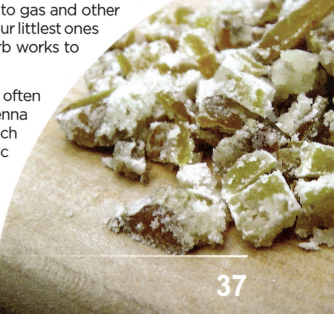

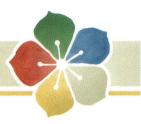

Dried Orange Peel

Most of us eat the fruit of an orange and throw the rest away. In doing so we are throwing away the most nutritious part! Chinese medicine has used a variety of citrus peels for thousands of years. In Traditional Chinese Medicine, dried orange peel is used to "transform" phlegm in the Lungs or the Spleen and to drain dampness. From a western perspective we can consider this herb when we want to ignite our metabolic fires and promote digestion.

FOR THIS RECIPE YOU'LL NEED...

- 1 tablespoon minced candied ginger
- 1 tablespoon dried orange peel powder
- 3 tablespoons fennel seeds

First mince the candied ginger.

Measure out your fennel seeds.

Measure out the orange peel powder.

And then mix them all together.

We keep this delicious mixture on our dinner table in an airtight container. We eat about a teaspoon or more after meals.

You'll notice that this is a small recipe. Feel free to make this in much larger batches!

EXERCISE, CARMINATIVE

Explore Carminative Herbs

Carminative herbs are a fun group to study. Since these are our most delicious herbs, they are pleasure to immerse yourself in.

The following are some ideas on how to freshen up your relationship to these delightful spices.

Clean out your spice cabinet!

Throw out old spices that have lost their kick and replace them with more vibrant herbs and spices.

Seek out new spices

Did you notice any spices in the carminative presentation that you've never tried before? Or maybe some familiar herbs that you've never tried in cooking? (Like lavender?) Pick one new thing and try it out!

Try some different cuisines

There are many traditional cuisines from around the world that actively use LOTS of herbs and spices in their dishes. Learning these recipes can be a fun and flavorful way to experience the taste of herbs! We love cooking Indian food at our house. Thai, Mexican, Chinese, French, Ethiopian, Spanish and so on. Share your favorite recipes in our community forums. If everyone shared one favorite recipe we would have quite the collection!

Further Resources

Here are the two books I listed in the presentation. If you have favorite books about spices or favorite cookbooks that use lots of spices please share them in our community forums!

Healing Spices by Bharat B. Aggarwal

The Three Sisters Indian Cookbook: Flavours and Spices of India by Sereena Kaul, Priya Kaul, Alexa Kaul

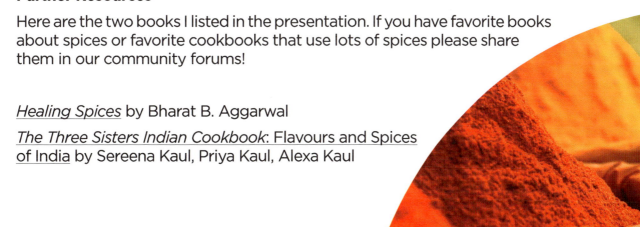

EXERCISE, CARMINATIVE

Kitchari

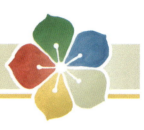

Kitchari is the comfort food of India. It's considered a balancing meal that can promote health and wellness. It's often referred to as the "soul food" or "chicken soup of India. Kitchari is frequently recommended as a simple food for a person recovering from illness or for a modified fast.

Before we get started let's look at our ingredients more closely.

Basmati rice

Basmati rice is a wonderfully fragrant species of rice. The word basmati roughly means aromatic in the Hindi language. It's been cultivated in India for thousands of years, and is a highly sought-after grain due to its delicious flavor. Although I buy a lot of my grains from bulk bins, basmati rice is much fresher and better tasting when sold in a closed container.

Mung Beans

Mung beans are originally from India and are also a traditional therapeutic food in China. According to Paul Pitchford, in his book Healing with Whole Foods, they are often used for cooling and draining the body specifically in times of damp heat such as summer heat, diarrhea, red rashes with swelling, edema of the lower extremities, gastro-intestinal ulcers, and dysentery. Mung beans are specifically considered beneficial to the liver and gallbladder.

To increase the digestibility of dried beans, I like to soak them about 5-7 hours along with some whey or yogurt. Soaking dried beans breaks down indigestible sugars in the beans, resulting in less gas, and it also allows for a shorter cooking time.

The spices...

Cumin (*Cuminum cyminum*)

Cumin is perhaps one of the first herbs ever cultivated. It is warming and slightly bitter and often used in cooking to promote digestion. It increases circulation, dispels gas, and can quell nausea. It was used in Ancient Egypt as medicine, as well as in the embalming process. The Bible references the use of cumin, also.

Coriander (*Coriandrum sativum*)

Coriander seeds come from the cilantro plant. It is another herb that has been used for literally thousands of years. It's considered to be hot and pungent like many of our "culinary" spices often used to promote digestion. Herbalist Brigitte Mars says that coriander seeds can be used topically to relieve cramps, neuralgia, and to stop hemorrhoidal bleeding.

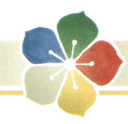

Turmeric (Curcuma longa)

Turmeric is currently our featured herb at HerbMentor. Instead of asking what this amazing rhizome can do, it would be far easier to ask what it can't do. A potent anti-inflammatory as well as a digestive aid, turmeric is commonly used for all sorts of ailments, including chronic pain, gastric ulcers, regulating blood sugar, and stopping fungal infections.

This recipe calls for ghee or coconut oil. I avoid using olive oil when cooking and prefer these more stable oils. Ghee is clarified butter and can be bought at health food stores or easily prepared at home.

TO MAKE THIS RECIPE YOU'LL NEED......

- 1 cup of basmati rice
- 1/2 cup of mung beans (or other types of legumes such as lentils)
- 2 tablespoons of whey or yogurt
- 2 & 1/2 cups of water
- 1 onion
- 2-4 tablespoons coconut oil or ghee
- 1 tablespoon turmeric
- 1 tablespoon coriander
- 1 tablespoon cumin
- 1/2 teaspoon ground pepper
- 1 teaspoon salt or to taste

Step one (in advance)

Begin by looking over the mung beans for any stones or other debris. Once they have passed inspection, soak the mung beans overnight or in advance with the whey or yogurt.

When you are ready to start cooking, strain the beans and rinse them well along with the rice.

Place the rinsed rice and beans in a pot with 2 and a 1/2 cups of water.

Heat on high until it starts to boil. Reduce heat to low and continue to let it simmer for 30 minutes.

Ten minutes before the rice and beans are

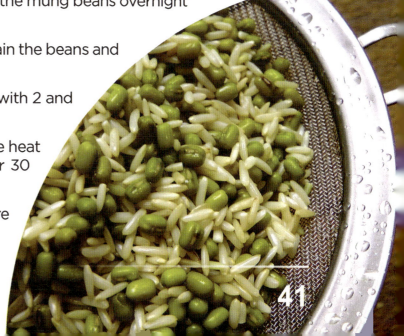

finished cooking, heat coconut oil or ghee in a large pan.

Add chopped onions to the warmed oil and saute until they become translucent.

Add the spices and saute for about 30 seconds or until you start smelling the spices.

Add the cooked rice and mung beans mixture and combine the two together well.

Variations

This above recipe is very simple and is very amenable to variations.

The different spices that could be used in this recipe are endless. Some others you may want to try include cinnamon, cardamom, bay leaves, ginger, etc.

Try quinoa instead of basmati rice.

Any variety of vegetables can be added to the rice and beans.

I especially like adding a lot of cilantro.

More broth can be added to make it more of a soupy texture.

Coconut milk and/or shredded coconut can add an additional flavor.

EXERCISE, CARMINATIVE

Les Herbes de Provence

I used to think Les Herbes de Provence was some ancient French tradition, but it turns out this term was just a marketing technique pulled out in the 1970s.

Nevertheless, these blends do feature herbs that famously grow throughout the Provence region.

Use this blend to flavor just about anything! Grilled meats and fish, veggies, and stews are delicious with this blend. When I lived in France, my favorite sandwich shop used an herbes de Provence blend on their sandwiches—delicious! Even works well as a tea.

I like to make this up in bulk so that it's always on hand when I need it.

WHAT YOU'LL NEED...

- 1 part savory
- 1 part thyme
- 1 part basil
- 1/2 part lavender flowers

Combine all the herbs and store them in an airtight container in a dark location.

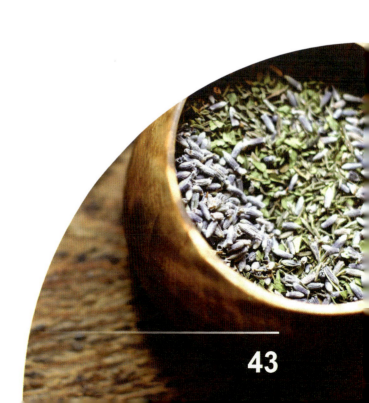

EXERCISE, CARMINATIVE

Parsley Pesto

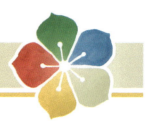

Parsley is often left behind on restaurant dinner plates, but that one small leaf is probably the most nutritious thing on them! Parsley is full of nutrients, most notably antioxidants that are being studied in their role against cancer.

We love to make this pesto all year long. In the summer our garden supplies ample amounts of parsley, and we can still find parsley in the grocery store during the colder months. You can also freeze this for later use.

WHAT YOU'LL NEED...

- 2 cups tightly-packed flat-leaf parsley leaves
- 3/4 cup toasted chopped walnuts
- 1/2 cup grated Parmesan cheese
- 3 large cloves garlic, crushed
- 1/2 teaspoon salt
- 1 teaspoon paprika powder
- 1 cup extra-virgin olive oil
- 2 tablespoons fresh lemon juice
- 2 teaspoons lemon zest

Throw everything in a food processor and blend until smooth.

Use liberally on meats and veggies.

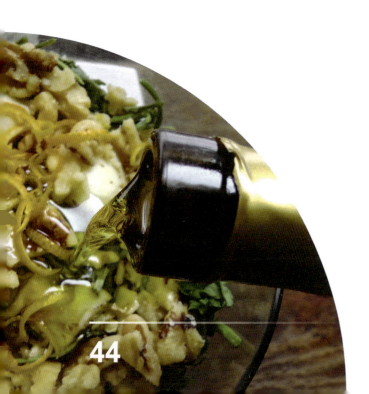

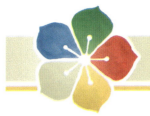

EXERCISE, RELAXING NERVINE

Comparing Basils

When people learn about Holy Basil or Tulsi, they often ask if culinary basil can be used in the same way. In fact, that's a common question in general: Can this herb be used for that herb?

A great way to explore the similarities and differences between plants is through taste. Does it taste similar on your tongue? Does it feel similar in your body?

In this exercise, we are comparing Tulsi (*Ocimum sanctum*) to our more common basil (*Ocimum basilicum*). It's preferable to use fresh basils for this, but dried works well too. If you come across fresh basils later, consider trying this again.

WHAT YOU'LL NEED...

- 1 tablespoon dried or 2 tablespoons fresh holy basil
- 1 tablespoon dried or 2 tablespoons fresh culinary basil
- 16 ounces of just-boiled water
- masking tape, pen
- two identical mugs

Use the masking tape and pen to mark the identical mugs. One is for holy basil, the other is for culinary basil.

Make the tea, letting it steep for 10 minutes. Strain and make sure you get the tea in the right cups.

Mix the cups around until you don't know which one is which.

Taste each cup of tea. Notice the different tastes. Notice and record the differences in both taste and how they make you feel. Remember there are no wrong answers, you're making observations.

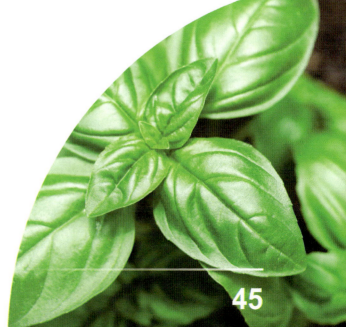

EXERCISE, RELAXING NERVINE

Nutmeg Milk

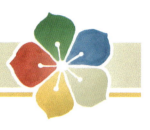

This is a classic drink to help induce a deep slumber. Nutmeg is a wonderful relaxing nervine, but take care with the dosage. Take just the right amount and you'll sleep through the night. Take a bit too much and you'll feel groggy the next day. Take waaaay too much (like an ounce) and you'll get a nasty reaction or sort of high that teenagers try once in a while, which then makes the headline news. Nutmeg isn't dangerous, just pay attention to the dose!

Nutmeg is, by far, the best when freshly ground. You can buy special grinders for nutmeg. I just use the smallest grinder such as a cheese grater. Once it is ground it loses its umph rather quickly (within days), so it's best to just grind as much as you need from whole nutmeg rather than buying it pre-powdered.

WHAT YOU'LL NEED...

- 8 ounces of warmed milk or milk substitute
- 1/2 teaspoon of freshly ground nutmeg
- 1 tablespoons of rose water (optional)
- honey to taste

Warm the milk gently, being careful not to scald it. Once warmed, add the nutmeg and let it sit for five minutes covered.

Add the rose water and honey. Stir well.

Drink 1-2 hours before bedtime.

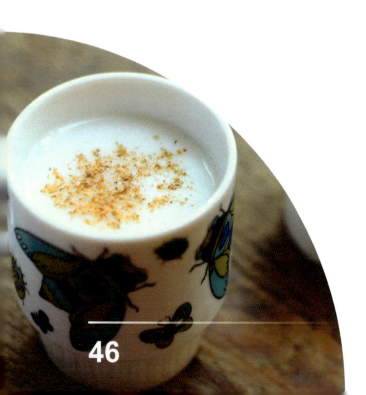

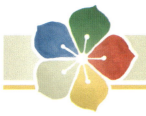

EXERCISE, SIALAGOGUE

Mouthwash

This mouthwash is highly antimicrobial and a sialagogue. It can be used 2-3 times a week to maintain mouth health. Or it can be used 2-3 times a day (20 minutes swishing each time) for more acute problems.

Keep in mind that mouth infections can be very serious. If left untreated the infection can spread to the brain and become fatal. See a dentist or visit the ER if you have a mouth infection that is not responding to at-home treatments.

WHAT YOU'LL NEED...

- 1/2 ounce Echinacea tincture
- 1/4 ounce Oregon Grape Root tincture
- 1/8 ounce Plantain tincture
- 1/8 ounce Spilanthes tincture
- 1-2 drops peppermint extract, optional (if using essential oils they MUST be from a very reputable source)

To use this blend, simply combine the above amounts in a 2 ounce amber bottle with a dropper.

Then place 30-60 drops in a mouthful of water. Swish for 5-20 minutes and spit out the mixture.

When swishing for longer periods of time, you may need to periodically spit out a bit of the liquid since it will be gradually increasing with the added saliva.

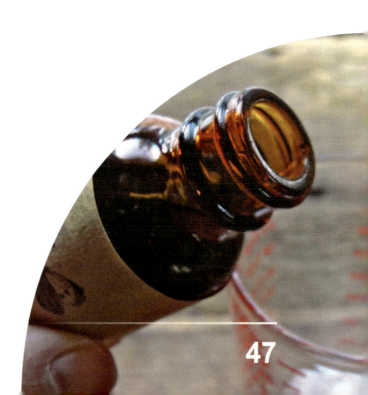

EXERCISE, STIMULATING DIAPHORETIC
Cayenne Tea

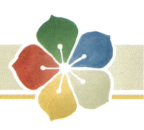

Get ready to sweat! Cayenne is an incredibly diffusive herb that almost immediately pushes fluid out of the skin, hence sweating! Taking a hot cayenne tea (or hot ginger tea) is one of the first things I do when I feel a cold or flu coming on. Not only does this speed the healing process and shorten the duration of a cold or flu, it also feels really good on the throat (ironically).

The first time I made cayenne tea it wasn't pretty. Don't do what I did and try to make this with a tablespoon of cayenne powder. Holy smokes! If you have really potent cayenne powder, then start with just an 1/8 or 1/4 teaspoon. If you can handle that well, then slowly increase the amount. The hotter the better, but you will get nauseous if you drink something that is too strong for your tummy. My last advice is to sip this slowly. Again, it can upset the belly if you drink it too fast.

WHAT YOU'LL NEED...

- 1/4 tsp cayenne powder (more or less)
- 1 tablespoon lemon juice
- 1 teaspoon of honey (or to taste)
- 8 ounces of hot water

Place the cayenne powder in a cup. Pour the just-boiled water over it. Stir.

Add the lemon juice and honey. Stir. Sip slowly once it has cooled. The hotter you drink this the better.

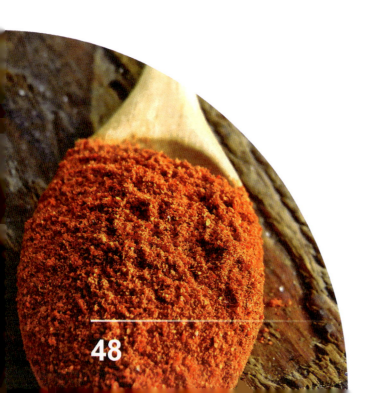

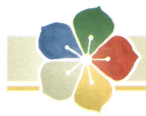

EXERCISE, STIMULATING DIAPHORETIC

Tom Kha Soup

Tom Kha soup is a dish from Thailand. It might possibly be my most favorite dish ever. The richness of the coconut milk mingles with the tartness of the lemongrass in a base of super delicious bone broth soup. It just tastes so darn good!

We make a big batch of this soup once a week and eat it numerous times throughout the week. When we have dinner guests or bring food to folks (because of injury or recent birth), we generally serve this soup. And we always hear people ranting and raving about it.

We love to eat this soup in the winter time as part of our medicine cabinet to keep our immune systems strong throughout the winter and to avoid getting upper respiratory infections like a cold and influenza.

It's packed full of powerful immune herbs and spicy warming herbs that are perfect for the cold winter months. This is also a quite spicy dish. You'll see. It will make you sweat!

There are lots of Tom Kha recipes out there. I hope you enjoy this version, which has a few more local veggies than what you'll typically see in these recipes. Soups beg to be altered, so experiment away!

Before we get to the recipe here's a bit more information about the yummy herbs in this soup and the health benefits in it...

Lemongrass

Lemongrass is a prominent spice in Thai cooking. It has an aromatic, lemony scent and taste, but it also has something more. I find it hard to describe myself, but I recently heard someone describe it as a lemony pepper taste with a hint of rose.

Besides its seductive taste, lemongrass is a powerful medicinal herb. It's used for fevers, digestive complications, and headaches.

It makes a delicious tea. I often add small amounts to other tea blends simply because I love the taste of it so much.

The oil of lemongrass is referred to as citronella which is commonly used as an insect repellent.

This recipe calls for fresh lemongrass. If you can't find it fresh, you can also make a strong tea out of dried lemongrass for a similar taste. I would try two heaping tablespoons of lemongrass in 8 ounces of just-boiled water. Let it sit for 10 minutes, then strain and add the water to the soup.

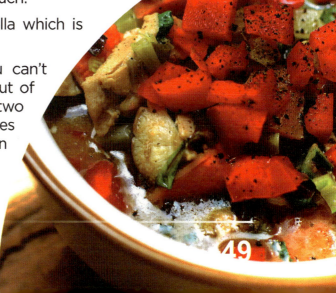

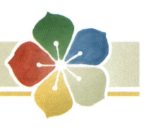

Cilantro

Cilantro is often thought of as simply garnish for guacamole, but this is yet another unassuming plant that is disguised as potent medicine.

Before I go on, I know someone out there is thinking, "Yuck! I hate cilantro." It's true people seem to either adore cilantro or detest it. If you think cilantro tastes like soap, then it's probably not your fault! Some people genetically lack the ability to taste the flavor that most people love in cilantro. Concurrently they also have a stronger reaction to another flavor within cilantro. If you don't like cilantro, feel free to omit it from the soup.

Cilantro is loaded with antioxidants. It's an aromatic carminative herb that's great for promoting digestion. My teacher Michael Tierra recommends strong cilantro tea or cilantro pesto for stubborn urinary tract infections.

Garlic

Garlic is a strong antimicrobial herb that stimulates circulation and boosts the immune system. Just eating one fresh clove a day (not the bulb) can deliver powerful health benefits such as supporting good cholesterol ratios and promoting digestion.

Ginger

Ginger is a spicy herb that can promote digestion, quell nausea, lessen headaches, reduce pain, fight intestinal infections, and shorten the duration of a cold or flu. Ginger is one of my most reached for herbs simply because it does so much and it does it so well!

Shitake Mushrooms

I adore shitake mushrooms, so I love piling them in the soup until it looks like I am eating shitake mushroom soup! Shitakes are a wonderful food for the immune system. They have been studied extensively for preventing and treating cancer.

WHAT YOU'LL NEED...

- 32 fluid ounce bone broth
- 3 cans regular coconut milk (look for BPA free coconut milk)
- 2 big stalks lemongrass, sliced in large pieces
- 4 tablespoons fish sauce
- 2 tablespoons low sodium soy sauce
- 2 tablespoons apple cider vinegar
- 4 tablespoons lime juice

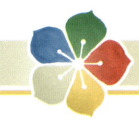

- 4 tablespoons minced ginger
- 8 cloves minced garlic
- 1 pack skinless chicken thighs, cubed in very small pieces (sometimes we use salmon instead)
- 8 ounces shitake mushrooms, sliced
- 1 bunch bok choy, chopped
- 1 bunch of kale chopped
- 1 bunch green onions
- 2 carrots, chopped
- 1 tablespoon green thai curry paste
- 1 bunch fresh cilantro, chopped (leave the stems in!)

Directions:

Heat the bone broth and coconut milk in a large, heavy bottomed pan.

Once the liquids are heated you can add the fish sauce, tamari, apple cider vinegar, lime juice, ginger, and garlic.

Bring the broth to a slow simmer. Make sure it doesn't boil and do not cover it during cooking.

When the broth is simmering, add the chicken, mushrooms, bok choy, kale, green onions, carrots, and green curry paste.

When the chicken is fully cooked and the carrots are tender, add the cilantro. After a minute, taste the soup and add some lime juice, if desired.

It's ready to serve! A cilantro and red pepper garnish is a nice touch.

This recipe makes a lot of soup. Perhaps 8 - 12 servings. It makes great left overs!

EXERCISE, STIMULATING DIURETIC

Diuretic Tea

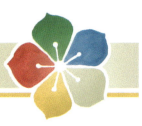

Here is an example of a diuretic tea that uses stimulating and irritating diuretics. It's safe for most people to use and can give you a taste (literally) of how diuretics work. If you have any special medical issues (heart medication, diuretic medication, etc.) it would be best to skip this exercise.

This recipe combines pungent, sweet, and bitter herbs. When tasting it try to tease those tastes apart.

WHAT YOU'LL NEED...

- 3-6 juniper berries crushed
- 1 teaspoon marshmallow root
- 1 teaspoon yarrow leaves and flowers
- 8 ounces just-boiled water

Place the herbs in a cup and cover with the just-boiled water.

Let it steep for 30 minutes. Strain and drink lukewarm to cool.

For extra credit try drinking this hot and then later cool. What differences do you notice?

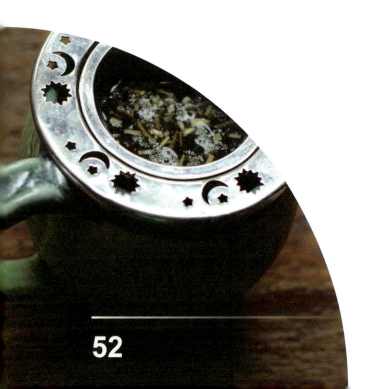

EXERCISE, PUNGENT

Juniper with Caramelized Apples and Onions

When used sparingly, juniper is an interesting pungent taste. It works well in meat marinades and makes a delicious dessert, which was inspired by the folks at the365kitchen.com.

WHAT YOU'LL NEED...

- 1 tablespoon butter or ghee
- 2 medium-sized tart apples, sliced thinly
- 1/2 of a medium onion sliced thinly
- 10 crushed juniper berries
- 2 sprigs of rosemary
- 3 cloves of garlic
- 1 teaspoons of lemon juice
- salt and pepper to taste

Heat the butter on medium heat.

When the butter is melted, add in the apple, onion, crushed juniper, and rosemary.

Cook on medium heat, stirring frequently to prevent burning. When onions turn translucent, throw in the garlic cloves whole so they roast and soften.

Continue to stir frequently (about 12-15 minutes) until onions and apples are caramelized.

Season with salt and pepper.

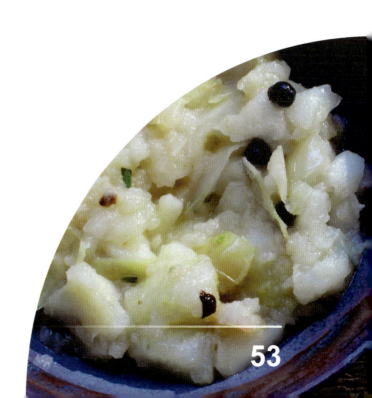

EXERCISE, STIMULATING EXPECTORANT

Elecampane Honey

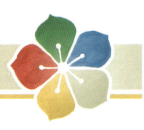

This is a staple at our house for those wet boggy coughs. The honey is soothing to an inflamed throat and elecampane is a fabulous stimulating expectorant.

If you don't have access to fresh elecampane root, consider growing it. It's so gorgeous in the garden. You can also order fresh roots from small herb farms. If the dried root is really all you have then make a simple syrup instead.

WHAT YOU'LL NEED...

- fresh elecampane root, minced
- local raw honey
- jar

Fill your jar half of the way with the minced elecampane root. (Don't forget to taste that root! It's a memorable experience.)

Next fill the jar with your high quality honey. Stir and fill again, if necessary.

Let this sit for a minimum of three days to many months. We leave the elecampane root in the honey and chew it up.

Over time, the honey may crystallize, but it will last for a very long time.

To use this for productive coughs, adults take one tablespoon every hour or a teaspoon every 1/2 hour.

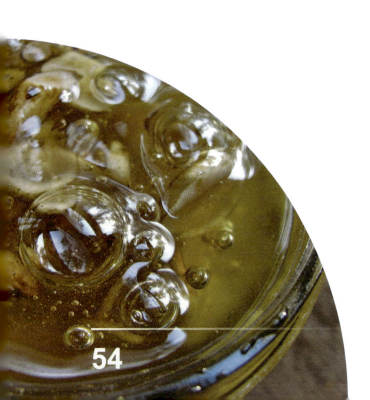

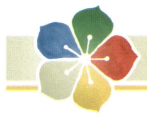

EXERCISE, STIMULATING EXPECTORANT

Fire Cider by Erin McIntosh

Mmm...mmm...How I love this hot and sweet, zesty, vinegary recipe! Fire Cider is a traditional cold remedy with deep roots in folk medicine. The tasty combination of vinegar infused with powerful immune-boosting, anti-inflammatory, anti-bacterial, anti-viral, decongestant, and spicy circulatory movers makes this recipe especially pleasant and easy to incorporate into your daily diet to help boost the immune system, stimulate digestion, and get you nice and warmed up on cold days.

Because this is a folk preparation, the ingredients can change from year to year depending on when you make it and what's growing around you. The standard base ingredients are apple cider vinegar, garlic, onion, ginger, horseradish, and hot peppers, but there are plenty of other herbs that can be thrown in for added kick. This year I had lots of spicy jalapenos and vibrant rosemary in the garden, so I used those along with some organic turmeric powder and fresh lemon peel. Some people like to bury their fire cider jar in the ground for a month while it extracts, and then dig it up during a great feast to celebrate the changing of the seasons.

Fire Cider can be taken straight by the spoonful, added to organic veggie juice (throw in some olives and pickles and think non-alcoholic, health-boosting bloody mary!), splashed in fried rice, or drizzled on a salad with good olive oil. You can also save the strained pulp and mix it with shredded veggies like carrots, cabbage, broccoli, and fresh herbs to make delicious and aromatic stir-fries and spring rolls! I like to take 1 tablespoon each morning to help warm me up and rev the immune system, or 3 tablespoons at the first sign of a cold.

WHAT YOU'LL NEED...

- 1/2 cup fresh grated organic ginger root
- 1/2 cup fresh grated organic horseradish root
- 1 medium organic onion, chopped
- 10 cloves of organic garlic, crushed or chopped
- 2 organic jalapeno peppers, chopped
- zest and juice from 1 organic lemon
- several sprigs of fresh organic rosemary or 2 tablespoons of dried rosemary leaves
- 1 tablespoon organic turmeric powder
- organic apple cider vinegar
- raw local honey to taste

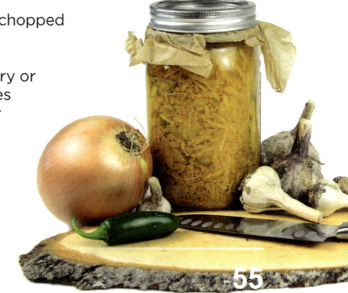

Directions

Prepare all of your cold-fighting roots, fruits, and herbs then place them in a quart jar. If you've never grated fresh horseradish, be prepared for a powerful sinus-opening experience! Fill the rest of the jar with the vinegar. Use a piece of natural parchment paper or wax paper under the lid to keep the vinegar from touching the metal. Shake well! Store in a dark, cool place for one month and remember to shake daily.

After one month, use cheesecloth to strain out the pulp, pouring the vinegar into a clean jar. Be sure to squeeze as much of the liquid goodness as you can from the pulp while straining. Next comes the honey! Add 1/4 cup of honey and stir until incorporated. Taste your cider and add another 1/4 cup until you reach the desired sweetness.

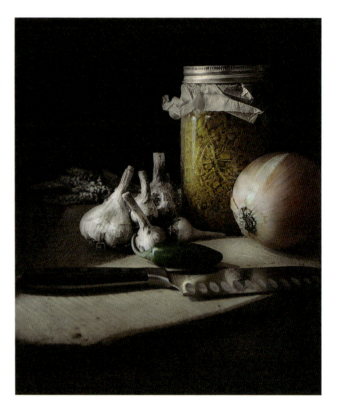

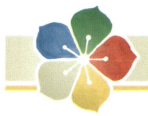

EXERCISE, STIMULATING EXPECTORANT

Homemade Mustard

A couple years ago my husband and I were traveling through France to visit our family. The trip had gone absolutely perfect until about the last week there when I caught a cold.

I quickly went through the small tincture bottles I had brought with me and was still a stuffy, foggy-headed mess. Even though it was just a little cold, I felt miserable! I really wanted to get the most out of every second in France, so I was desperate for something to help me.

I was standing in the kitchen of my husband's aunt and uncle's house, bemoaning my stuffy sinuses, when I suddenly realized that there was an forgotten but very potent herb that is found in practically every French kitchen: Mustard!

Sure enough, I found several different kinds of mustard in the fridge and took a spoonful of one of them.

Holy smokes!

Mustard, especially well-prepared authentic mustard, is pungent, spicy, and downright hot!

My sinuses immediately started to drain and I started to sweat. I kept up with my regular dosings of mustard, and I was feeling a lot better in no time.

Mustard's Powerful Healing Abilities

The power of mustard goes far beyond a simple cold and flu!

Allyl isothiocyanates (AITC) are compounds found in mustard seeds that have been studied extensively for their ability to prevent and decrease cancer cells. There are over 200 studies showing these positive effects!

Mustard seed and oil have also been shown to protect heart health by reducing inflammation and normalizing cholesterol levels.

Using a mustard seed poultice has been a long-lived folk tradition to help people with congested lung mucus and bronchitis. It's also been shown to reduce symptoms of COPD.

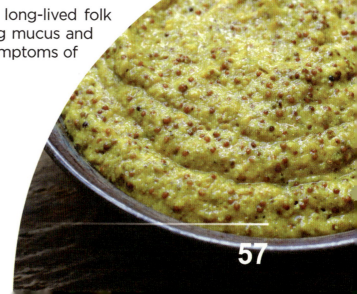

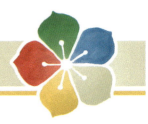

Why Make Your Own Mustard?

Making your own mustard is really simple and super cheap. By avoiding store-bought brands you are also avoiding common artificial flavors and colorings.

When you make your own mustard you can create many different herbal varieties.

Different Kinds of Mustard Seeds

There are two kinds of mustard seeds that are readily found in commerce: yellow and brown.

Yellow mustard seeds have a milder flavor and brown mustard seeds have a much hotter and spicier flavor. The following recipe uses both yellow and brown mustard seeds, but if you prefer a milder taste use only the yellow.

This recipe is super simple but takes a few days to complete. The mustard seeds need to be soaked in water and apple cider vinegar for two days to let the flavor of the mustard seeds release.

Here's what you'll need to make this recipe

INGREDIENTS...

- 1/4 cup brown mustard seeds
- 1/4 cup yellow mustard seeds (use only yellow seeds if you want a milder taste)
- 1/2 cup apple cider vinegar
- 1/2 cup water
- 1 teaspoon honey
- 1 teaspoon turmeric powder
- 1 teaspoon salt

Place the mustard seeds, apple cider vinegar, and water in a glass bowl. Cover and let sit for about two days.

When the mustard seeds are through soaking, place them, as well as the liquid, into a food processor or blender.

Add the rest of the ingredients and blend until the mustard is ground into a paste.

This recipe makes about a pint of mustard. It will keep in the fridge for about six months.

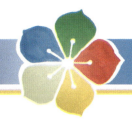

SALTY

Ayurveda Elements

Earth and Fire
heavy, hot and wet

TCM Organs

Kidney and Bladder
yin

Chemical constituents

Minerals, Sodium Chloride

How we use the salty taste

A salty taste can promote digestion, moisten the body, act as a laxative, relieve stiffness, and dissolve cysts.

Examples

A salty taste comes from minerals. It is found in salts, seaweeds, and irish moss. Herbs that have high mineral contents are seen as having a salty taste. These include herbs such as nettle *(Urtica dioica)* and cleavers *(Galium aparine)*.

Contraindications

Hypertension, edema (for pure salts, not mineral rich herbs).

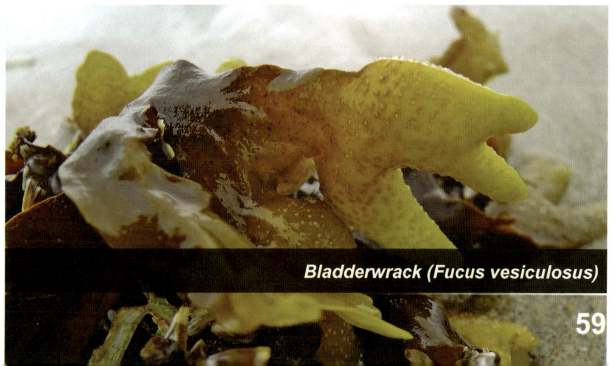

Bladderwrack (Fucus vesiculosus)

EXERCISE, SALTY INTRODUCTION

With and Without Salt

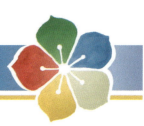

Not only is salt a valuable and necessary mineral for humans, we love the flavor it imparts to foods. How salt works to create flavor is pretty interesting.

Salt can enhance the umami or savory flavors. This is why a steak or soup without salt can taste dull, but just a bit of salt then brings the dish to life. Salt increases the aromas or smell of foods, and the smell of a food enhances its taste as well.

Salt can add a depth of taste to sweet foods. This is why it is added to sweet baked goods.

Just a bit of salt can modify a bitter taste, also.

In this exercise you can see these aspects of salt for yourself.

EXERCISE #1

WHAT YOU'LL NEED...

- What you'll need...
- one grapefruit
- salt

Slice the grapefruit in half. On one half lightly sprinkle salt. Leave the other half plain. Taste one and then the other. What difference do you notice?

EXERCISE #2

WHAT YOU'LL NEED...

- 1 tomato (preferably in season and home grown but any will do)
- salt

Slice the tomato. Lightly sprinkle some salt on one slice and leave another slice without salt. Taste one and then the other. What difference do you notice?

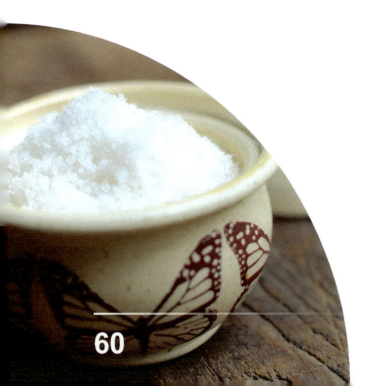

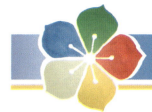

EXERCISE, NOURISHING HERBS

Apple Cider Vinegar Infused with Chickweed

In this recipe, apple cider vinegar helps to extract all the minerals from the nutrient-dense chickweed. The vinegar can then be used in your favorite salad dressing or other culinary recipes.

Although vinegar extractions have a predominantly sour taste, I wanted to add them to the nourishing herbs exercises because vinegar extract minerals really well. (And as we've learned, many of the benefits of nourishing herbs come from the mineral content.)

Alcohol, on the other hand, doesn't extract vitamins and minerals making alcohol tinctures a poor choice for nourishing herbs.

INGREDIENTS

- apple cider vinegar
- minced chickweed
- jar (with a plastic lid or some sort of barrier to protect the metal from corrosion)

To begin, simply fill a jar with loosely-packed chickweed.

Cover this with apple cider vinegar.

Place a plastic lid on the jar, or put wax paper in between the liquid and the metal lid. (Vinegar will corrode metal over time and ruin the mixture.)

Shake this for a few moments each day for four weeks.

After four weeks (you can wait longer, if desired), strain off the vinegar and use it as desired.

The "marc" or chickweed can be composted.

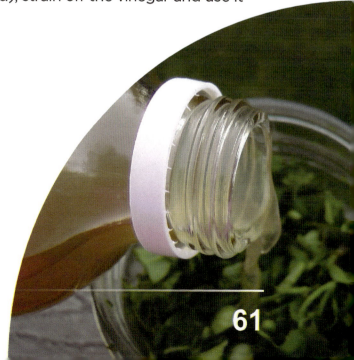

EXERCISE, NOURISHING HERBS

De la Forêt Salad Dressing

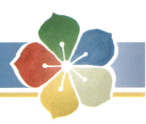

This salad dressing contains all the flavors! The sour taste of the vinegar, the salty taste of the miso, the pungent spicy herbs and mustard, and the savory taste of the olive oil with a dash of honey for sweetness.

We eat it on salads, salmon, and with artichokes.

WHAT YOU'LL NEED…

- three tablespoons of olive oil
- one tablespoon apple cider vinegar (an herbal-infused vinegar is best)
- one teaspoon of mustard
- one teaspoon of miso
- one clove of garlic crushed
- one teaspoon of herbs such as thyme, oregano, parsley, basil, etc.
- one teaspoon of honey

Mix all the ingredients together, stirring until blended.

We can make this in a small batch so that we'll use it within a day or two.

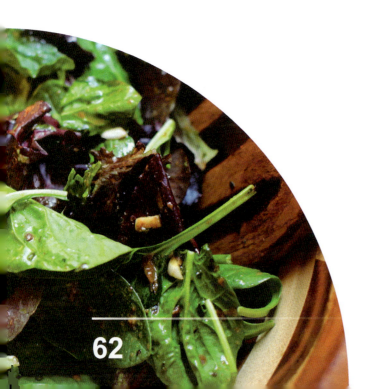

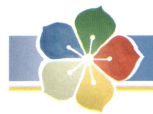

EXERCISE, NOURISHING HERBS

Kale Chips

We may not often think of kale as an herb, but I think it rides a thin line between herb and vegetable. Like nettles, kale is full of nutrients and has a slightly bitter and salty taste.

WHAT YOU'LL NEED...

- three tablespoons of olive oil
- one tablespoon apple cider vinegar (an herbal-infused vinegar is best)
- one teaspoon of mustard
- one teaspoon of miso
- one clove of garlic crushed
- one teaspoon of herbs such as thyme, oregano, parsley, basil, etc.
- one teaspoon of honey

In a large bowl, combine the olive oil, apple cider vinegar, lemon juice, and salt. Mix well.

Take a large bundle of frizzy kale (about 10 leaves), destemmed, and cut it into bite-size pieces (roughly 2x2 inches). Toss the kale in the olive oil mixture, making sure all the leaves are coated well without being soaked.

Put the kale in a large baking dish or on a cookie sheet. Bake at 350 degrees for 10-12 minutes. Then flip the kale and return to the oven for another 10-12 minutes or until the kale is slightly crispy but not burnt.

Serve immediately.

This amount makes a side dish for two people.

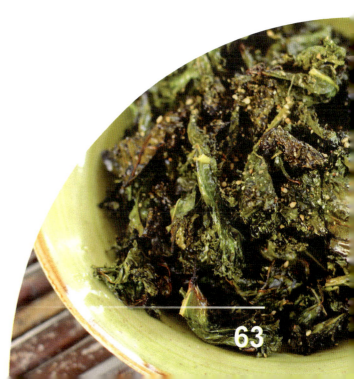

EXERCISE, NOURISHING HERBS

Oatstraw Tea

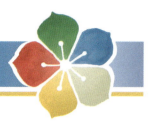

This is a favorite tea blend that I especially love serving to large crowds, which everyone seems to like!

The oatstraw contains a lot of mineral and is quite nourishing. The elderberries and rose hips give a pleasingly tart or sour taste to the tea. I often serve this tea simply as a pleasant-tasting tea, but it could also be viewed as a supportive immune system booster.

WHAT YOU'LL NEED...

- 20 grams oatstraw
- 10 grams rose hips
- 5 grams elderberries
- a pinch of stevia (or add honey to taste)
- one quart of water

Place the herbs and water in a stainless steel or glass pan.

Bring to a boil then reduce heat and simmer for 20 minutes.

Remove from heat and strain. Serve hot.

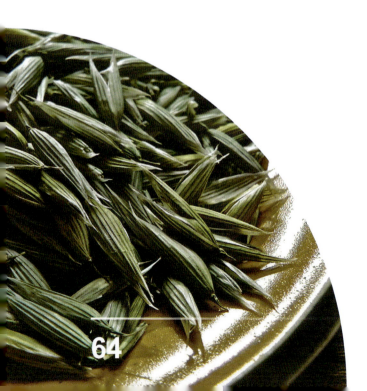

EXERCISE, NOURISHING HERBS

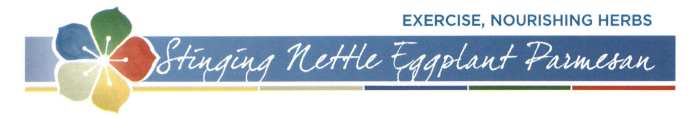

Stinging Nettle Eggplant Parmesan

This is a gluten free lasagna in which the eggplant becomes the noodles. I've been making this recipe for at least a decade, and it is very adaptable to your own preferences.

If you don't have fresh nettle, substitute a big handful of dried nettle, kale or other leafy greens.

Experiment and enjoy!

WHAT YOU'LL NEED...

- 1 diced onion
- 4 cloves of garlic, minced
- olive oil
- 2 16-ounce cans of crushed tomatoes or 2 pounds of fresh tomatoes (best to use your own preserved tomatoes or search out brands that do not contain harmful chemicals in the cans)
- 1 pound of cooked ground meat or sausage
- 2 large eggplants
- 1 bunch of fresh basil
- 2 tablespoons dried oregano
- 1 pound of fresh stinging nettle (Or a big bunch of kale and a handful of dried nettle)
- 2 cups grated mozzarella cheese
- 1/4 cup parmesan cheese
- salt and pepper to taste

Pre-heat oven to 325.

Slice eggplants lengthwise and lightly cover both sides with olive oil.

Place them on a cookie sheet. Do not overlap.

Bake them in the oven for 12 minutes and then flip over. Bake for 10 minutes more or until they are translucent in the middle. Set them aside.

Raise the oven temperature to 350.

Fill a large pot with water. Bring to a boil and add the fresh stinging nettle leaves. Boil for about 10 minutes and then strain well. Reserve the nettle water for drinking or for a rich fertilizer.

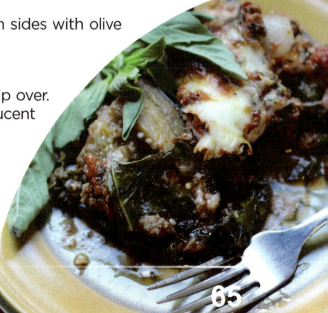

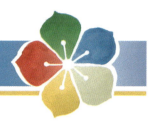

Meanwhile, in a large skillet or sauce pan, sauté onion in the olive oil until translucent. Add the garlic and sauté for a minute more (being careful not to overcook the garlic). Add the crushed tomatoes, the cooked meat, basil and boiled/strained stinging nettle. Let simmer for 15 minutes.

In a large casserole dish place a layer of the eggplant, followed by a thick layer of the tomato mixture, and a sprinkling of the cheeses. Continue this until the ingredients are used up or there is no more room in the casserole dish.

Bake in the oven at 350 for 25-30 minutes or until it is slightly browned and heated through. Let it cool before serving.

EXERCISE, NOURISHING HERBS

Violet infused oil

Violets have long been praised for their ability to soften lumps. They are a gentle herb that can move stagnant tissues and bring health to areas rich in lymphatic tissue.

I frequently recommend this blend to support breast tissue health. It can be gently rubbed into the breasts and arm pit areas every day.

WHAT YOU'LL NEED...

- fresh violet leaves and flowers
- dried calendula flowers
- oil of your choice

Fill the jar half full with the fresh violet leaves and flowers. Fill it another quarter full with dried calendula flowers.

Fill the jar with an oil of your choosing. Olive oil is nice and stable, but has a greasier feeling than jojoba, almond or grape seed oil. Stir well.

Cover the jar.

Open the jar every day for the next two weeks and stir the contents. Fresh herbs in oil can easily spoil if you forget about them! Place the jar in a place where you'll easily see it as a reminder. Ideally this place will be cool and dark.

After two weeks strain off the oil. If desired, you can add a few drops of lavender essential oil to the mixture.

Use it daily to support healthy breast tissue and remove stagnation.

Note: This mixture can help move stagnant lymph. It's not a treatment for cancer.

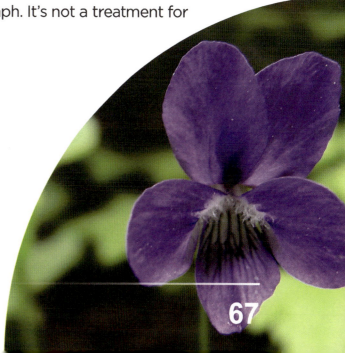

EXERCISE, SALT

Artisanal Salts

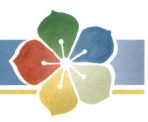

Here is a brief listing of the various gourmet salts that you can purchase. There is a whole world of culinary salt appreciation out there!

My local health food store carries all of these salts. You can find them at Mountain Rose Herbs or other online retailers.

FRENCH SEA SALT

This is my favorite salt. I keep a small jar of it on the table and add a tiny pinch of this flaky salt as a finish to my meals. Regular table salt doesn't dissolve well after cooking so adding salt just before eating can lead to adding too much salt in order to compensate. French sea salt dissolves readily and imparts a sweeter salty taste. It is perfect for adding post cooking. My husband prefers things less salty, so this allows us both to be happy.

RED ALAEA SALT

This salt comes from Hawaii and is treated with the local clay. This imparts a deep red color due to iron deposits in the area. It has a delicate taste and goes well with veggies.

BLACK LAVA SALT

This salt has been treated with charcoal and is especially high in nutrients. It has a stronger flavor that goes well with grilled food and meats.

PINK HIMALAYAN SALT

Harvested from the Himalayan mountains, this salt is often considered to be more pure and free from chemical pollutants than can be found in sea salts. It contains numerous trace elements.

REAL SALT

I was born and raised just miles from this salt mine in Utah. This salt is very comparable to pink Himalayan salt in terms of minerals, but it's more "local" and a lot cheaper. This is the salt we use for every day cooking.

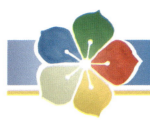

SMOKED SALT

As you might imagine, smoked salts impart a smoky flavor to foods. It's best to use this in small amounts and use another salt if additional salty taste is needed. I like this sprinkled on top of chocolate.

EXERCISE, SALT

Bath Salt Blend

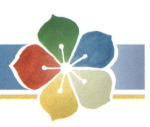

Bath salts can be a luxurious gift and they can also be a powerful tool to help ease aches and pains. When people ask me what they should take after overdoing it physically, epsom salt baths is always one of my first answers! I can't tell you how many times I've sunk sore muscles into a hot bath of epsom salts and found relief from pain.

Sometimes bath salt recipes have small amounts of salts to the bath. I add a lot of salts to the bath because it is much more therapeutic. Experiment with amounts and see what you like best.

WHAT YOU'LL NEED...

- 1/2 cup baking soda
- 2 cups epsom salts
- 1 cup sea salt
- essential oils (optional)

Mix all the ingredients together in a large bowl.

Using a spoon or whisk, blend in the essential oils. I frequently use lavender, sage, rosemary and/or peppermint in my bath blends. I use anywhere from 20-40 drops for this quantity of salts.

Once blended, store the salts in an airtight container. The above recipe makes one bath.

Optional:

If you are making this for a gift (or if you like pink as much as I do), add just a tablespoon or two of pink Himalayan salt or red alaea salt to add a splash of color to the blend.

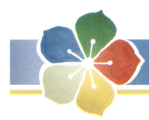

EXERCISE, SALT

Celery Salt

Celery salt is a delicious salt seasoning that can be added to just about everything including soups, sandwiches, meats and veggies. It's a common ingredient in coleslaw.

The recipe is listed in parts. You can make this in whatever quantity you desire. For example you could do 1 tablespoon celery seed and 2 tablespoons salt. Or 1 cup celery seed and 2 cups salt.

WHAT YOU'LL NEED...

- 1 part celery seed
- 2 parts finely grained salt (I like Redmond Real Salt)

Grind the whole celery seed into a fine powder. (Be sure to taste the celery seed by itself. How would you describe the taste?)

Mix it with the salt.

Voila!

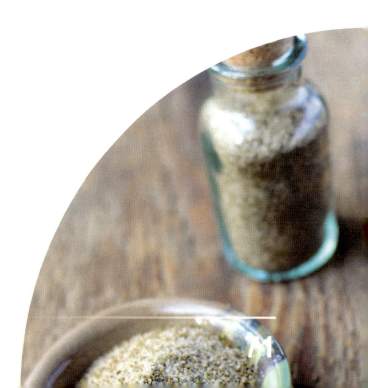

EXERCISE, SALT

Chamomile Popsicles

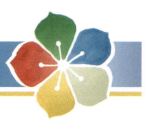

This fun popsicle recipe that tastes great and is great for rehydrating the body on a hot summer day. It includes the essential ingredients for rehydration including water, salt, and sugars; plus, the benefits of two wonderful herbs.

Chamomile is truly an amazing herb. It can soothe a distressed child (or adult!), calms tummy troubles, and provides support during colds and flus. This all-purpose herb is safe for children and kids who love a sweet and mild taste.

Hibiscus flower is high in vitamin C and has a great tart taste. It also has the added benefit of turning these popsicles pink!

Besides helping to rehydrate the body, they can also be used for children (and adults) who are recovering from any kind of stomach illness such as diarrhea, upset tummy, or even vomiting. Chamomile can soothe the entire digestive tract, and the yogurt is a good source of probiotics.

WHAT YOU'LL NEED...

- 2 tablespoons of dried Chamomile
- 1 tablespoon of dried Hibiscus
- 1 and 1/4 cup boiling water
- 1 cup of greek yogurt
- honey to taste
- a pinch of salt
- 1 tablespoon of lemon juice
- popsicle molds (You can use paper cups and popsicle sticks)

Begin by making a tea out of the chamomile and hibiscus. Put the herbs in a cup, pour the water over the herbs, and let it steep for 5 minutes.

Strain into a small bowl.

While the mixture is still hot, add honey to taste. Stir well so the honey combines with the tea. You will be mixing this with the plain yogurt, so you may want to make it more on the sweet side.

Add a pinch of salt.

Add the lemon juice. You can use the juice of a fresh lemon. We keep this type of fresh lemon juice on hand for convenience.

Let the mixture cool a little.

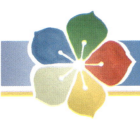

Add the yogurt and mix well.

Pour into the popsicle molds.

Place these in the freezer until frozen solid. This will take several hours.

This recipe is just one example of how to make herbal popsicles. There are many different herbs you could use as well. There are also a variety of different ingredients you could use. For example, you could try adding a mashed banana or rose hips.

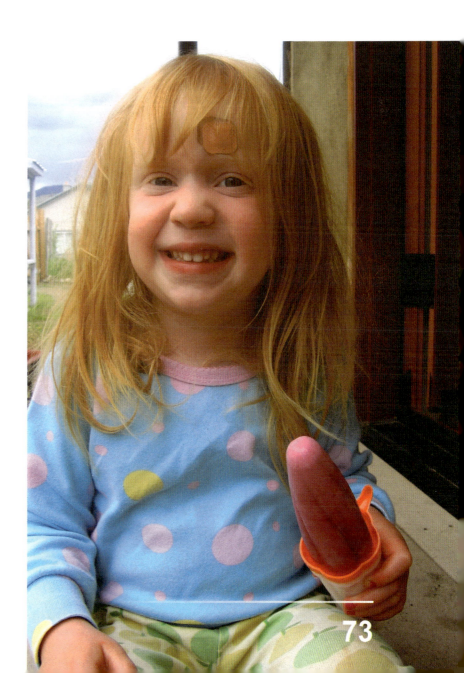

EXERCISE, SALT

Saline rinse for eyes and nose

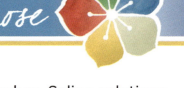

This is a simple saline wash to use for neti pots or eye washes. Saline solutions help to soothe irritated eyes and mucus membranes. They're a lot more gentle than using water alone.

Neti pots are an Ayurvedic tool for washing out the sinuses. They are best used when there is dryness in the sinuses and not when there is congestion.

Eye cups can be purchased at most pharmacies and can be used for eye infections (like conjunctivitis) or other eye irritations.

Here are some special considerations when making your saline solution.

Use distilled water. Tap water can contain chlorine, fluoride, and other chemicals that are not eye/nose friendly.

Be as sterile as possible. Wash all instruments with hot soapy water and consider boiling them before use.

If you are addressing an eye infection, sterilize the eye cup in between eyes so you avoid spreading the infection to the other eye.

WHAT YOU'LL NEED...

- 1/2 teaspoon salt (sea salt or real salt; avoid using table salt)
- 1 cup distilled water
- 1/4 teaspoon baking soda (optional for nasal rinses)

Bring the water and salt to boil in a pan. Boil for five minutes. Let it cool.

Use the solution in a sterile neti pot or eye cup. This solution needs to be made daily.

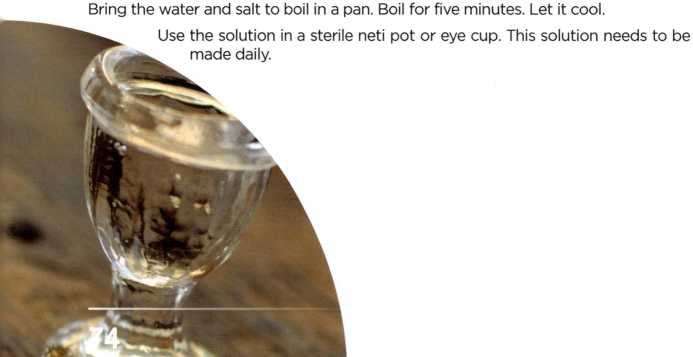

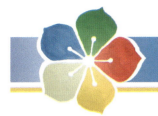

EXERCISE, SALT

Salt Scrub

Salt scrubs are a mixture of salts and oils. This mixture is gently massaged into the skin. This exfoliating treatment helps remove dead skin cells and promotes lymphatic movement.

I like to use a really fine grain of salt for my salt scrubs, but others may prefer a coarser grain. (A finer grain will be less abrasive for sensitive skin.)

A variety of different oils can be used. Olive oil is a thicker oil that will feel more oily on the skin. Almond oil and grape seed oil are less oily but still nourishing. Rose hip seed oil is fabulous for damaged skin.

You can also vary the amount of oil in the recipe for a more or less oily salt scrub.

This recipe uses calendula infused oil which results in a gorgeous orange scrub. You can buy or make your own calendula infused oil or substitute another infused oil.

WHAT YOU'LL NEED...

- 1 & 1/2 cups sea salt
- 1/2 cup calendula infused oil
- 1/4 cup sesame oil
- 40 drops grapefruit essential oil
- 30 drops lavender essential oil
- 30 drops fir essential oil

Dampen the skin (I rinse off in the shower, then turn the water off).

Using your hand or a shower mitt gently rub the salt into the skin. I start at the feet and work my way up using circular motions.

Avoid wounds, varicose veins, and other sensitive areas of the skin.

Rinse well and prepare to be amazed at your glowing soft skin!

EXERCISE, SALT

Simple Electrolyte Blend

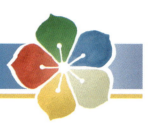

I learned this simple electrolyte blend from Dr. Aviva Romm many years ago and have used it for myself and others numerous times. It can be especially important when there is an increased risk for dehydration including vomiting, diarrhea, fevers, or excessive sweating.

Dehydration is a potentially dangerous condition. Seek out emergency medical care if the situation necessitates it.

WHAT YOU'LL NEED...

- 1 quart of water
- 1/2 teaspoon of salt
- 1/2 teaspoon of baking soda
- 2-3 tablespoons of honey or sugar
- juice of half a lemon

Mix all the ingredients together (you may need to heat the mixture slightly to get everything to blend well). Drink it in frequent sips.

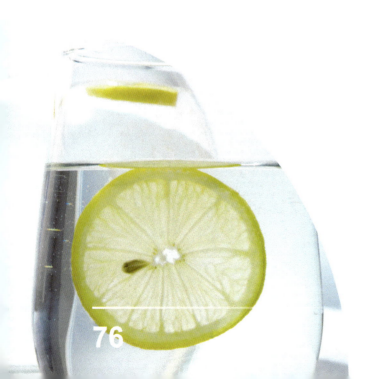

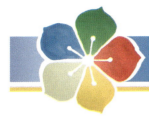

EXERCISE, SEAWEED

Salmon and Seaweed Soup

This is a tasty soup that everyone will love. It is especially suited to our section on salty taste, not only because of the seaweed, but also because of the salty miso and fish sauce. Vegetarians can omit the fish sauce and salmon and increase the salt and vegetables. Like most soups it's a versatile recipe.

This recipe does not taste like seaweed. For those more habituated to the taste of seaweed you may want to add a bit more seaweed to increase the benefits.

WHAT YOU'LL NEED...

- 2 pounds salmon filets, cut into 1-inch cubes
- 4 tablespoons olive oil
- 3 medium onions, finely sliced
- 4 cloves garlic, minced
- 1 tablespoon minced fresh ginger
- 2 large carrots, chopped
- 2 tablespoons fish sauce
- 2 quarts water or soup stock
- 1 tablespoon lemon juice
- 1 large bunch of kale, chopped
- 1 teaspoon fermented miso (per person)
- Seaweed: 1/4 teaspoon kombu flakes, 1/4 teaspoon macro flakes, 1/4 teaspoon wakame flakes (per person)
- Parsley to garnish

In a large skillet, heat the oil, and add the onions on medium-high heat. Cook until translucent. Reduce heat to medium.

Add the garlic, ginger, and carrots, and cook until the carrots are just tender.

In a large pot with 2 quarts of water (or soup stock), add the salmon, onion, carrot mixture, fish sauce, and cook on medium-high for about 10 minutes until the salmon is just cooked.

Remove from heat. Add the lemon juice and kale.

In individual bowls, add the miso and seaweed; plus, add a little broth and mix until the miso is dissolved, then add the rest of the soup. Garnish with parsley, if desired.

Makes about 6 servings.

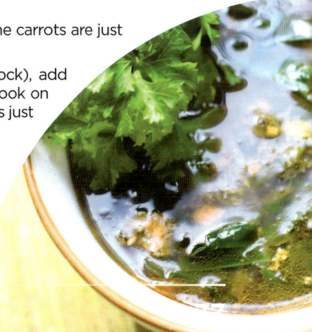

EXERCISE, SEAWEED

Seaweed Bath

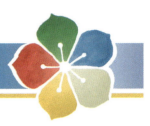

Many of the health benefits of seaweed can be experienced through baths! In fact, seaweed baths have historically been a popular therapeutic remedy in European spas. Even today many high-end spas offer seaweed wraps and baths.

You can create your own luxurious seaweed experience at a fraction of the cost of fancy spas. Consider adding salts too!

WHAT YOU'LL NEED...

- 1/2 cup to 1 cup dried seaweed. I recommend kelp or wakame.
- mesh bag
- hot water and a bath tub (or use it as a foot soak)

Place the dried seaweed into the mesh bag. The seaweed will swell in size once it absorbs the water, so put it in a larger bag. Make sure the bag is tightly closed.

Add the bag to the bath water. When you squeeze the moistened bag, you'll feel it ooze a demulcent gel. I like to spread this over my skin and face.

Soak in the hot seaweed bath for 20 minutes or longer.

You can dry out the seaweed bag and use it again or add it to your compost.

Tip: If you are buying seaweed for your bath, many small seaweed companies offer B grade seaweed that is cheaper than their primo stuff. I buy the A grade for eating and B grade for baths.

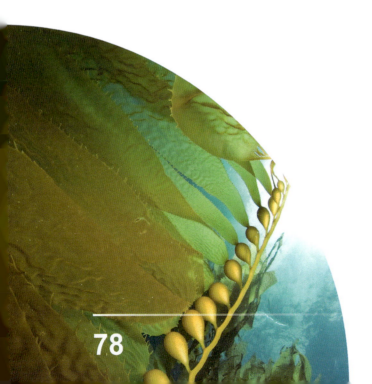

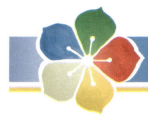

EXERCISE, SEAWEED

Seaweed Cookies

I first learned this basic recipe from ethnobotanist Karen Sherwood. This is truly a favorite treat at our house. I love to bring it to potlucks because it can inspire some interesting conversations.

Even if you think you don't like seaweed, give these a try. They are delicious.

If you can't eat nuts, try these with roasted sesame seeds instead.

WHAT YOU'LL NEED...

- 1/4 cup of granulated kelp (Nereocystis luetkeana)
- 2 & 1/2 cups of ground nuts (I often blend almonds and walnuts)
- 1/2 cup of maple syrup
- Coconut oil (or butter) to oil the pan

Blend together the granulated kelp and ground nuts.

Add the maple syrup. The end consistency should be a sticky dough that isn't too wet.

Grease a 9X9 glass casserole dish using coconut oil or butter.

Transfer the mixture to the casserole dish. With clean, wet hands, evenly press the nut mixture into the dish.

Bake at 350° for 15-20 minutes. It's done when the center no longer looks moist and the edges are golden brown.

Let it cool and cut it into bars.

HERE ARE SOME ADDITIONAL VARIATIONS:

- shredded coconut
- dried fruits
- chocolate chips
- nettle seeds

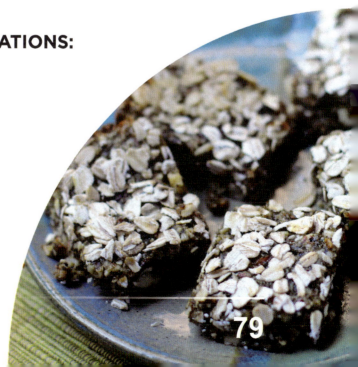

EXERCISE, SEAWEED

Seaweed Salt Scrub

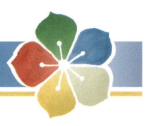

I love having ridiculously soft skin. Like the kind of skin that gets compared to a baby's butt. I also love indulging in a spa experience in the comfort of my own home! This recipe accomplishes both of these!

WHAT YOU'LL NEED...

- 1 tablespoon powdered kelp
- 1 tablespoon powdered rose petals
- 1/8 cup fine to medium ground salts (fine for more sensitive skin)
- 4 tablespoons French Green Clay
- Olive oil
- 15 drops lavender essential oil (optional)
- 3 drops vetiver essential oil (optional)

Mix together the kelp, rose petals, clay, and salts.

Pour in about 3 tablespoons of olive oil. Mix well. Add a bit more olive oil. Stir well.

Keep adding and stirring in the olive oil until the mixture is a gloppy and slurry to use your sea scrub.

This makes enough for one body scrub. Start with a couple tablespoons of the mixture on your fingertips and rub into your dry skin in a circular motion.

Keep applying the mixture until you are completely covered. You may want to avoid sensitive skin areas such as a rash or delicate areas.

If desired, let it sit on the skin for 10-20 minutes. You can keep rubbing it in periodically.

Rinse well with hot water when finished. Careful, the tub may be slippery.

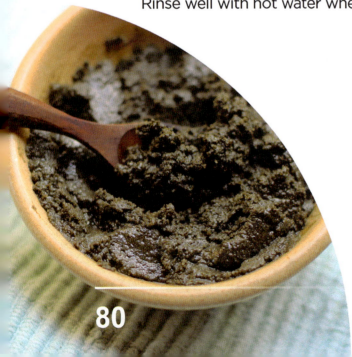

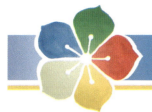

EXERCISE, SEAWEED

Sea Zest Seasoning

This recipe combines three sources of nutritional powerhouses for a tasty herbal seasoning that adds zest to vegetables, meats, sandwiches, salads, and possibly even ice cream.

The kelp and nettle are both considered to have a salty taste. If you put some kelp in your mouth, it definitely tastes salty. Nettle, however, doesn't have a definitively salty taste in the same way that kelp does. Because nettle is extremely high in minerals, it gets categorized as being in the salty taste category.

Sesame seeds are an excellent source of minerals like copper and manganese. They also contain a good amount of magnesium, calcium, iron, phosphorus, and zinc.

Kelp (Nereocystis luetkeana) contains a vast amount of nutrients. According to the authors of Vegetables from the Sea:

"All the minerals required for human beings, including calcium, sodium, magnesium, potassium, iodine, iron and zinc are present in sufficient amounts. In addition there are many trace elements in seaweeds."

Kelp also has significant amounts of vitamins A and C, as well as B1, B2, B6, Niacin, and B12. By adding this nutritious weed of the sea to our diets, we can find that our hair grows faster and thicker; and our bones, teeth, and nails are stronger. Seaweed supports metabolic function, also.

Stinging nettle leaf (Urtica dioica) is one of our most nutritious plants. According to Mark Pederson who wrote the book <u>Nutrional Herbology</u>, nettle contains high amounts of calcium, magnesium, chromium, and zinc.

Making this herbal seasoning is easy.

WHAT YOU'LL NEED...

- 1 & 1/2 cups toasted and ground up sesame seeds
- 1/2 cup dried granulated kelp (or use whole kelp fronds that have been processed into flakes)
- 1/2 cup dried nettle leaves

Step 1 ~ Preparing the sesame seeds

You can buy sesame seeds in packages or in bulk at your natural foods store. Sesame seeds are high in oils and can go rancid easily, so be sure to buy from a fresh source.

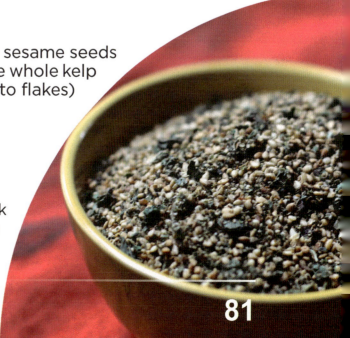

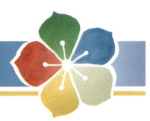

Toast the whole sesame seeds on low heat. We like to use a clean and dry cast iron pan for this, but whatever you have will work fine. Be sure to stir them often, so they toast evenly and do not burn. Once they become darker in color and have a nice aromatic smell, remove them from heat.

Using a food processor or blender, grind the seeds into powder and then place them in a large mixing bowl.

Step 2 ~ Mixing it together

Add one cup each of granulated kelp and cut-and-sifted nettle leaf to the sesame seeds.

If you are beginning with whole kelp fronds or a whole nettle leaf then you can use the food processor to mince them up. One word of caution is that it's better to have granulated kelp rather than powdered kelp. If it's too powdery, it doesn't mix well. Also, buying whole kelp fronds will ensure better quality than buying it granulated.

Once it is all mixed together you can bottle it up, label it, and enjoy!

Because sesame seeds are high in oils, you'll want to consume this seasoning quickly so that it doesn't have a chance to go rancid. If it has gone rancid, you'll notice the strong unpleasant smell.

You can store excess seasoning in the fridge for better storage.

This simple recipe can be a base for many other kinds of seasonings. You could add savory herbs like rosemary, thyme, or oregano. You could also add spicy seasonings like cayenne, ginger, or turmeric.

We sprinkle this seasoning on practically everything, but we haven't tried ice cream yet. Let us know if you do!

SOUR

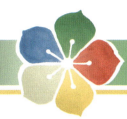

Ayurveda Elements

Water and Fire
hot, wet, and light

TCM Organs

Liver and Gallbladder
yin

Chemical constituents

acids, oxalic acid, citric acid, malic acid, vitamin C

How we use the sour taste

Sourness can increase digestive fire, increase strength, bodily tissues, counter thirst, promote healthy intestinal flora, and can be nourishing.

Examples

A sour taste can be found in fermented foods like miso, yogurt, berries, vinegar, and rose hips.

Contraindications

Burning sensations, hyperacidity, teeth sensitivity.

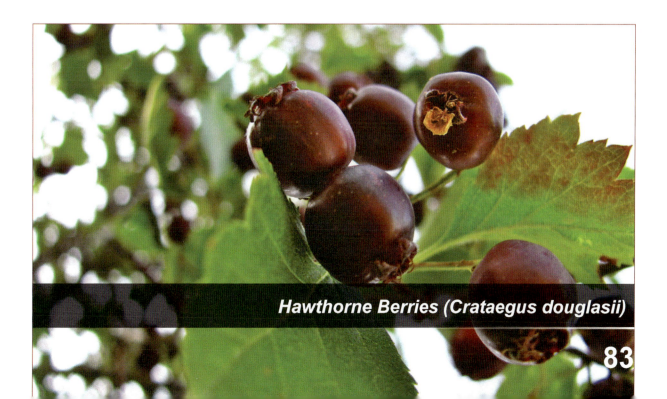

Hawthorne Berries (Crataegus douglasii)

EXERCISE, INTRO
Astringency Scale

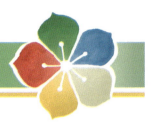

Astringency is the sensation you feel when you eat an unripe banana or drink a glass of red wine. It creates a puckering or drying sensation in the mouth.

In the pungent taste, we discussed how much pungent herbs can vary in energetics. Some are incredibly hot (like cayenne) while some are more moderate (like rosemary).

The same goes for astringent herbs.

The astringent action is really important in herbal medicine, and it's amazing how many herbs have the astringent herbal action.

But not all herbs listed as astringent have the same degree of astringency; therefore, we use these herbs differently.

We'll discuss astringency a lot more in the astringent video. But first, it's a good idea to understand the varying levels of astringent herbs. In this exercise, I encourage you to taste different astringent herbs and decide for yourself how astringent you think they are.

You can choose herbs you already have on hand by referring to the master list of astringent herbs. Here are the ones I particularly recommend trying. They can be tasted in any form, but I recommend trying just a bit of the powdered herb or making a simple tea out of them.

- oak bark
- rose petals
- uva ursi
- black tea
- green tea
- blackberry leaf/root

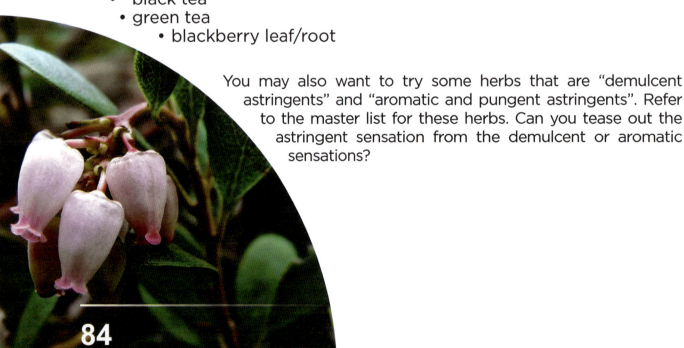

You may also want to try some herbs that are "demulcent astringents" and "aromatic and pungent astringents". Refer to the master list for these herbs. Can you tease out the astringent sensation from the demulcent or aromatic sensations?

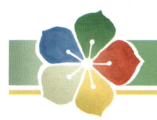

EXERCISE, INTRO

Lemon Water

Drinking a bit of lemon water in the morning is a folk remedy for supporting the liver and digestion. Some folks will have you believing it will cure anything that ails you. In Chinese Medicine, the sour taste is said to go to the liver. Give it a try and see what you think.

It's best to use warm or lukewarm water for this simple drink. Cold water inhibits digestion and should not be taken, especially with meals. Both TCM and Ayurveda agree on this. It's a strange thing that restaurants always serve iced water with a meal even in the middle of winter. Yikes! I always ask for water without ice.

WHAT YOU'LL NEED...

- 8 ounces of warm or lukewarm water
- 1 tablespoon of freshly squeezed lemon juice

Combine the two and sip in the time just after waking up, ideally before breakfast. Try it for a week. Do you notice any changes in your health? Does it help wake you up in the morning?

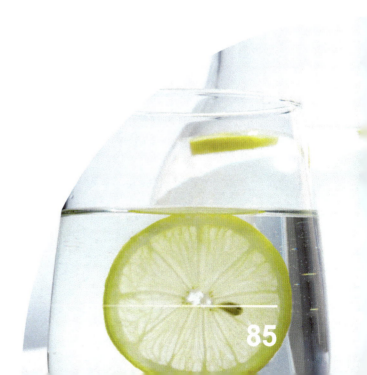

EXERCISE, INTRO

Sour or Bitter?

When I teach miniature versions of the Taste of Herbs to live classes, I notice that many people can't distinguish between sour and bitter. Both of these tastes, when really strong, can be unpleasant, and I think folks just equate these strong tastes as one thing.

I highly recommend you do the following exercise so that you are certain you know the difference between sour and bitter.

There's really no hard rule here. You just want to taste something that is decidedly sour and something that is decidedly bitter.

Here are some common foods and herbs to choose from.

SOUR
- lemons
- limes
- rosehips

BITTER
- dandelion leaves
- radicchio
- Brussels sprouts
- bitter salad greens

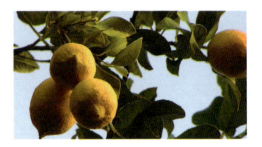

Once you know the difference between bitter and sour, you might taste different grapefruits; depending on the variety, many grapefruits are both bitter and sour. Can you tease apart the different tastes?

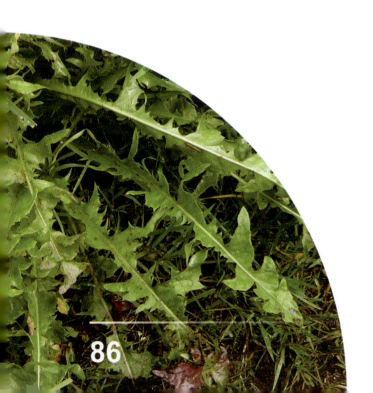

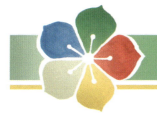

EXERCISE, ASTRINGENT

Bay Rum Aftershave

Aftershaves have a strong scent, but they do more than act as a cologne. They can also be used to protect the skin. When shaving, warm water is used to open the pores and soften the facial hair making it easier to shave. Aftershaves can be used after the shaving process to tighten and tone the pores on the face. This can prevent dirt and oil from entering the pores. This recipe is also anti-microbial, which can keep any razor cuts from becoming infected.

WHAT YOU'LL NEED...

- 2 cups of witch hazel extract
- 1 ounce of rum
- zest from one organic orange
- 1 cinnamon stick
- 3-5 cloves
- 3-5 whole allspice
- 1/2 teaspoon glycerin (optional)
- 1/2 teaspoon aloe vera (optional)
- Bay West Indies Essential Oil *(Pimenta racemosa)*
- Pint Jar

Begin by grating the orange peel to get its zest. You want the orange part of the peel, not the white beneath.

Once you have the zest, put it in your pint jar along with the cinnamon stick, the cloves, and the allspice.

Next, add the optional glycerin and aloe vera. These are great additions for sensitive skin.

Next, add the rum. You can buy a small one ounce bottle from the liquor store.

Next, fill the jar with witch hazel distillate. This will be just under two cups.

Finally, add 25-40 drops of the Bay West Indies essential oil.

Cover the mixture with a tight fitting lid and shake well.

Shake it well every day or so for 4-6 weeks.

Once it's done, strain off the ingredients and put it in a dark colored bottle. This makes enough to fill two 8 ounce bottles.

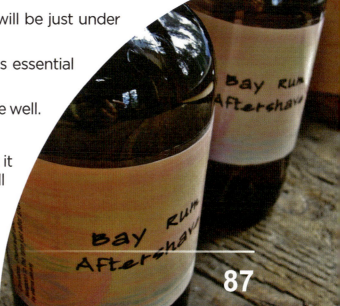

EXERCISE, ASTRINGENT

Facial Clay Mask

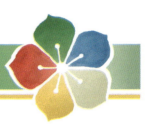

This recipe tightens and tones the pores of the face. It's perfect for oily skin. It's gentle enough for most skin types, also.

Clay is incredibly absorbent, while the astringency of rose petals helps tighten and tone the tissues. The lavender flowers are antimicrobial which is helpful for pimples on the skin. This facial mask can be used 1-3 times a week.

WHAT YOU'LL NEED...

To make a bulk blend use...
- 2 parts French green clay
- 1/2 part lavender flower powder
- 1/2 part rose petal powder

From that blend use...
- 1-2 tablespoons of the clay, rose, and lavender mixture
- 1-2 tablespoons of warm water
- 1 drop lavender essential oil (optional)

Mix the clay and water to create a smooth paste. Add more water if it's too thick or more clay if it's too loose. If desired, add one drop of lavender essential oil to this mix.

Apply the paste thickly to your face and leave it on for 10 to 20 minutes.

After rinsing the mask from your face, follow up with a splash of cold water.

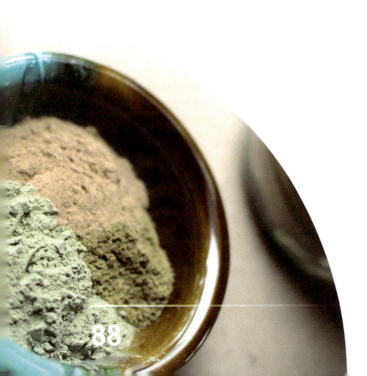

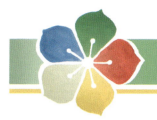

EXERCISE, ASTRINGENT

Facial Toner

This is a simple astringent facial toner that can be applied daily after washing your face and facial masks.

WHAT YOU'LL NEED...

- 2 ounces of witch hazel extract
- 2 ounces of rose hydrosol
- 7 drops of peppermint essential oil
- 7 drops of lavender essential oil
- 4 ounce spray bottle

Combine all the ingredients in the spray bottle.

To use, spray on face after cleansing or a facial mask.

This blend also feels lovely on hot days.

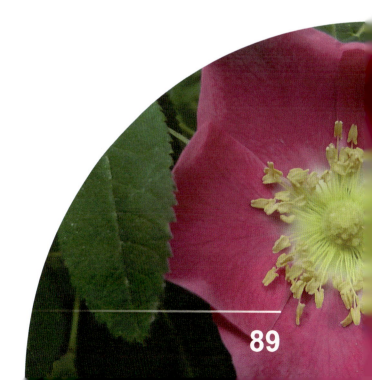

EXERCISE, ASTRINGENT

Leaky Gut Tea

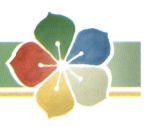

This tea blend combines the herbal actions of astringency, vulnerary (wound healing), and carminative. It heals the intestinal lining and promotes healthy digestion. It can be taken daily as needed.

If this blend is too cooling, a bit of ginger can be added to warm it up.

WHAT YOU'LL NEED...

- 10 grams plantain
- 10 grams goldenrod
- 5 grams calendula
- 5 grams meadowsweet
- 3-5 grams ginger (optional)

Combine the ingredients into a quart-sized mason jar.

Fill the jar with just-boiled water.

Steep for 30 minutes.

Strain and drink.

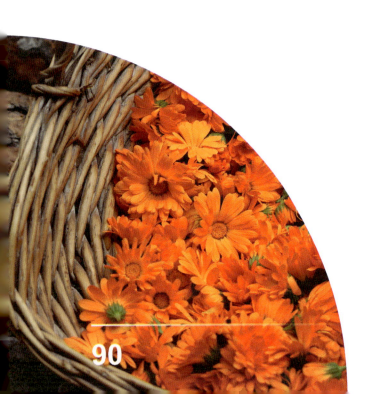

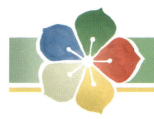

EXERCISE, ASTRINGENT

Mouth Pack

I learned this recipe and technique from Karta Purkh Singh Khalsa. I've used it with numerous people since with great results.

Turmeric and willow mouth packs are used to clear infection, as well as tighten and tone the gums. They will need to be applied at night for at least two weeks, and sometimes as long as 4 months in order to see results. Be sure to use a thick towel over your pillow at night as turmeric can stain.

WHAT YOU'LL NEED...

- 2 parts turmeric powder
- 1 part willow bark powder
- vitamin E oil (or water)

Mix the powders with either a tiny bit of vitamin E or water until it's moistened. Apply this to the gum line and leave it on overnight.

An alternative to this method is to place the moistened mixture in a gauze material and then place this along the gum line.

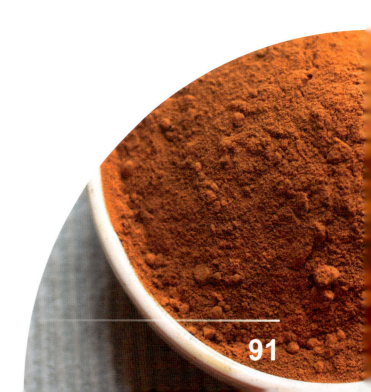

EXERCISE, ASTRINGENT
Rose Petal Vinegar

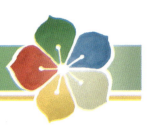

This is a lovely and simple recipe I first learned from Kiva Rose. I make this with fresh wild rose petals which bloom profusely all over our valley in June. I am also including a recipe for using dried rose petals in case you don't have access to fresh wild roses.

Some of you may be wondering if you can use domesticated roses. In general, I prefer wild roses for medicinal preparations. Domesticated roses are hybridized in order to achieve a special look. When this occurs, the more beneficial medicinal actions of the roses are diminished. You can always experiment to find out if your particular variety works. Avoid roses that have been sprayed with pesticides.

Whether you use fresh roses or dried roses, be sure to use a plastic lid or a plastic barrier between the metal lid and vinegar. Otherwise the vinegar will corrode the metal.

The vinegar tastes lovely and can be used in salad dressings. It can be very soothing to sunburns. To use it for sunburns, use 1/3 rose vinegar to 2/3 water and spray it on the affected area frequently.

WHAT YOU'LL NEED FOR FRESH ROSE PETAL VINEGAR...

- jar (your choice of size)
- fresh wild rose petals (enough to fill the jar gently packed in)
- apple cider vinegar
- plastic lid

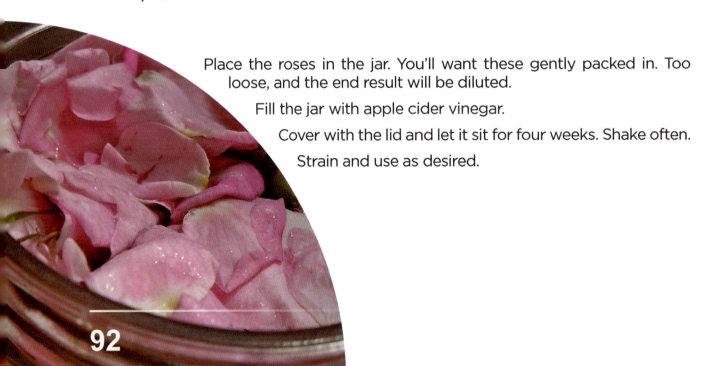

Place the roses in the jar. You'll want these gently packed in. Too loose, and the end result will be diluted.

Fill the jar with apple cider vinegar.

Cover with the lid and let it sit for four weeks. Shake often.

Strain and use as desired.

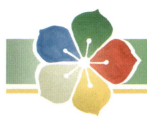

WHAT YOU'LL NEED FOR DRIED ROSE PETAL VINEGAR...

- jar (your choice of size)
- dried rose petals (enough to fill half the jar)
- apple cider vinegar
- plastic lid

Fill the jar half full with the rose petals.

Fill the jar with apple cider vinegar.

Cover with the lid and let it sit for 4 weeks. Shake often.

Strain and use as desired.

EXERCISE, ASTRINGENT
Simple Deodorant

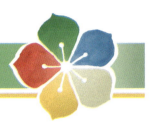

This is a super simple recipe for a deodorant that can be slightly antiperspirant, also.

Commercial antiperspirants are bad news. They clog your pores which inhibits your body's natural function of sweating. Sweating cools the body and gets rid of natural metabolic wastes. When we restrict this function with antiperspirants, it can actually cause us to sweat more.

If you use commercial antiperspirants, you may find that switching to a more natural deodorant, such as this one, will initially result in more sweating. But after a week or so this should decrease.

WHAT YOU'LL NEED...

- 2-ounce spray bottle
- 2 ounces of witch hazel extract
- 10 drops of juniper essential oil
- 10 drops of lavender essential oil
- 15 drops of grapefruit essential oil

Combine all the ingredients in a 2-ounce spray bottle.

Shake well before each use.

For especially hot days, you may find that this works best when reapplied a couple times throughout the day.

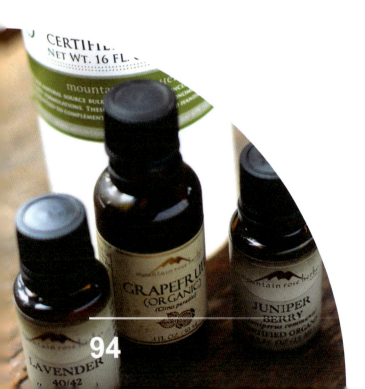

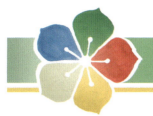

EXERCISE, ASTRINGENT
Sitz Bath

Sitz baths are a topical remedy used to heal wounds in the pelvic area. They are generally a combination of astringent and vulnerary herbs to inhibit infection and heal the wounds.

HERE'S WHAT YOU'LL NEED...

- 1 part calendula flowers
- 1 part rose petals
- 1 part plantain leaves
- 1 part uva ursi leaves

Mix the herbs together.

To make the sitz bath, use one cup of the herbs per quart of water.

Boil the water and pour over the herbs. Cover and steep for 30 minutes.

Strain. Use as a sitz bath for postpartum healing, hemorrhoids, or anal fissures.

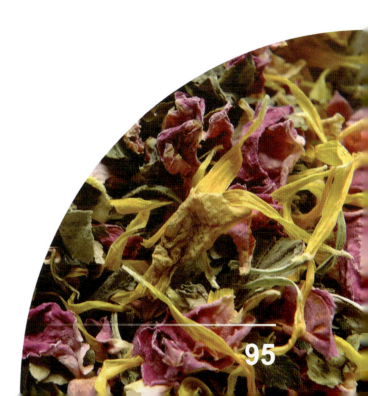

EXERCISE, ASTRINGENT

Uterine Tonic Tea

This is my favorite UTI (urinary tract infection) formula that works well for most UTIs.

For best results drink 1/4 to 1/2 cup every hour while symptoms are present. The amount can be decreased as symptoms decrease.

Yarrow is antimicrobial and diuretic.

Uva ursi is astringent, antimicrobial, and diuretic.

Marshmallow is soothing to the urinary tract and gut tissues.

Bee balm (or oregano) is antimicrobial and has a nice taste.

WHAT YOU'LL NEED...

- 10 grams yarrow
- 10 grams uva ursi
- 5 grams marshmallow root
- 5 grams bee balm (monarda fistulosa) or oregano

Combine the ingredients in a quart sized jar.

Fill the jar with just-boiled water.

Let sit for 30 minutes to 4 hours.

Strain and sip slowly. Do not add honey or sugar. You can alternate between this blend and unsweetened cranberry juice.

> This tea can cause nausea if taken in excess. If you start to feel queasy, decrease the dosage.

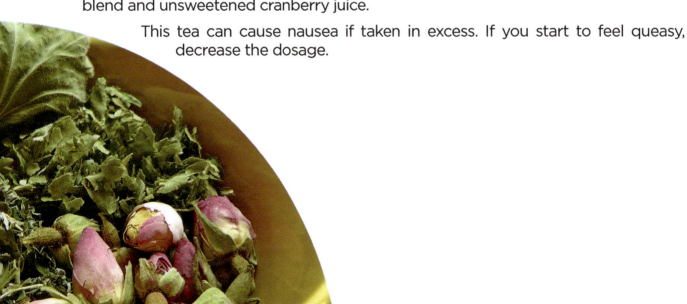

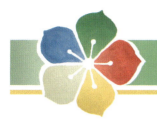

EXERCISE, ASTRINGENT

UTI Formula

This is my favorite UTI formula that works well for most UTIs.

For best results drink 1/4-1/2 cup every hour while symptoms are present. The amount can be decreased as symptoms decrease.

Yarrow is antimicrobial and diuretic.

Uva-ursi is astringent, antimicrobial and diuretic.

Marshmallow is soothing to the urinary and gut tissues.

Bee balm (or oregano) is antimicrobial and has a nice taste.

WHAT YOU'LL NEED...

- 10 grams yarrow
- 10 grams uva ursi
- 5 grams marshmallow root
- 5 grams bee balm (monarda fistulosa) or oregano

(THIS PAGE IS A DUPLICATE OF PAGE 98)

Combine the ingredients in a quart sized jar.

Fill the jar with just-boiled water.

Let sit for 30 minutes to 4 hours.

Strain and sip slowly. Do not add honey or sugar. You can alternate between this blend and unsweetened cranberry juice.

This tea can cause nausea if taken in excess. If you start to feel queasy back off a bit on the dosage.

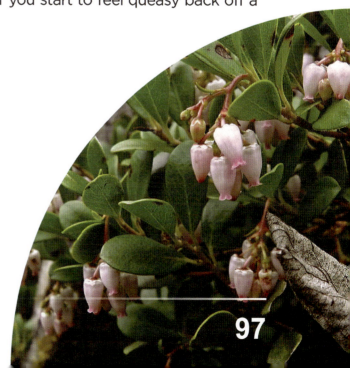

EXERCISE, ASTRINGENT

Varicose Vein Cream

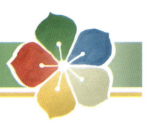

Varicose veins are essentially areas of stagnant blood. From an herbalist's perspective we want to address this condition by moving the blood and toning the tissues.

Calendula and yarrow move blood; plantain is healing and supportive to the tissues; while witch hazel, horse chestnut, and oak bark are astringent in nature helping to tighten and tone the tissues.

This recipe was inspired by Katja Swift.

HERE'S WHAT YOU'LL NEED...

- 20 grams of beeswax
- 25 grams of coconut oil
- 20 grams of shea butter
- 1/4 cup infused calendula oil
- 1/4 cup infused yarrow oil
- 1/4 cup infused plantain oil
- 1/3 cup witch hazel
- 1 ounce horse chestnut tincture
- 1 ounce oak bark tincture
- 40 drops of lavender essential oil (optional)

Melt the beeswax, coconut oil, and shea butter in a double boiler or on low until everything is melted. Remove from heat.

Add the infused oils. Reheat gently if necessary until the mixture is completely mixed together.

Let cool to room temperature.

Mix the witch hazel, tinctures, and optional essential oils together.

Place the cooled wax and butters mixture into a blender or food processor. Turn it on high.

Slowly drizzle the witch hazel and tinctures into the oils mixture, blending until the mixtures have emulsified and blended together.

Store this in a cool place. Use on varicose veins at least twice daily.

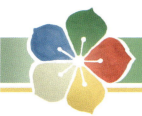

EXERCISE, BERRIES AND FRUIT

Hawthorne Cordial

In Chinese Medicine, hawthorne berries are used to stimulate stagnant digestion. In western herbalism, however, we use hawthorne berries to support heart health.

This blend adds the sweet and sour taste of fruit and honey to the pungent digestive spices of ginger, cardamom, and cinnamon. This is a wonderful blend for sipping after meals.

I was inspired to create this recipe after seeing a similar recipe from herbalist Juliet Blankespoor. This cordial is very amenable to substitutions. Experiment away!

WHAT YOU'LL NEED...

- 1 teaspoon minced fresh ginger
- 3 crushed cardamom pods
- 1 vanilla bean cut in half lengthwise
- 1 cinnamon stick
- zest from one lemon
- 1 fresh persimmon, chopped
- 1 apple, chopped
- 1/3 cup pomegranate seeds
- 1/2 cup dried hawthorne berries
- 2 tablespoons dried hibiscus petals
- 1/2 cup honey (or to taste)
- brandy

Place all of the spices and fruit in a quart-sized jar.

Add the honey and fill the jar with brandy.

Infuse this for 4 weeks. Shake often.

Strain.

Sip small amounts after meals to promote digestion.

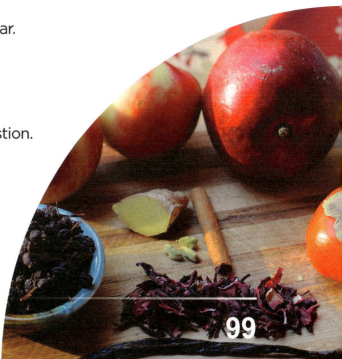

EXERCISE, BERRIES AND FRUIT

Limoncello

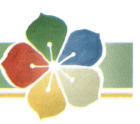

This tangy, one-hundred-year old recipe comes from the Amalfi Coast of Italy. It's an alcohol drink that's traditionally taken after a meal to promote digestion.

Limoncello is made in two steps: First, you (patiently) zest 11 or so lemons. I recommend using a vegetable peeler to slowly peel the lemon zest leaving the white pithy part behind. The zest will then be macerated in alcohol to make an extract out of it. (I've only made this with Everclear alcohol. If you don't have access to high proof alcohol, you could try vodka.)

This recipe only calls for the zest, not the juice of the lemons. Plan on making some spicy lemonade or some other recipe calling for lots of juice the day you start on this recipe.

The second part of this recipe is to combine a sugar syrup with the alcohol extract. I pride myself on giving out healthy, low sugar recipes, and this is by far the most sugar I've ever used in a recipe. You could try experimenting with less sugar, but the drink will not last as long. Keep in mind, this isn't exactly the healthiest drink. It's a great example of a sour herb being used to promote digestion.

WHAT YOU'LL NEED...

- zest from 11 organic lemons
- 1 quart of Everclear alcohol (150 or 190 proof)
- 1-3 cups sugar (Most recipes will call for 3 cups. I liked it around 2 cups)
- 3 cups boiling-hot water

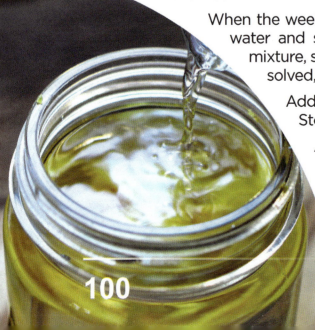

Put the lemon zest in a quart jar. Fill the jar with the Everclear. Let this sit for one week.

When the week is done start by making a sugar syrup. Place the water and sugar in a medium sized saucepan. Heat up the mixture, stirring frequently. Once the sugar is completely dissolved, remove it from heat and let it cool.

Add the alcohol mixture and sugar mixture together. Store in an airtight jar for two days.

After two days strain off the zest. The resulting liquid is your limoncello.

Serve 1-2 ounces chilled as an after dinner digestif.

Limoncello is often stored in the freezer or fridge. Use within six months.

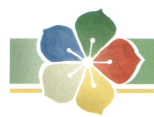

EXERCISE, BERRIES AND FRUIT

Pomegranate Molasses

This is a traditional Persian preparation that is used on sweet treats or drizzled onto savory meats and veggies. The taste is a delicious tangy sour flavor with a slight astringent aftertaste.

You can make this syrup from scratch by buying pomegranates and juicing the seeds. Call me lazy (go ahead, I can take it), but I prefer to simply buy the juice and reduce it into the syrup.

WHAT YOU'LL NEED...

- 1 pint of pomegranate juice
- 1 tablespoon of sugar

Combine the pomegranate juice and sugar into a small saucepan. Bring to a boil then immediately reduce to a simmer.

Simmer this until it has been reduced by 3/4 or until the mixture sticks to the back of a spoon.

Store in the fridge and use quickly.

We love this on vanilla ice cream.

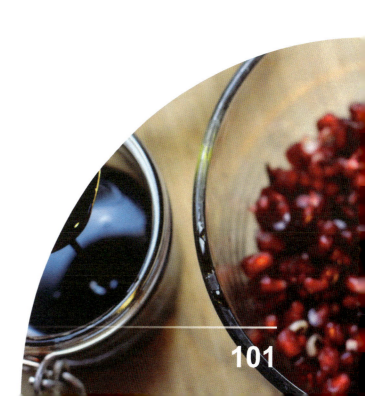

EXERCISE, BERRIES AND FRUIT

Rosehip and Cranberry Compote

I made this compote for my 5-year-old niece who proudly proclaimed, "Auntie Rosie makes the best cranberry sauce ever!" So, take it from my niece, Pearl. This recipe is yummy! (I should put her on the payroll.)

Cranberries are native to North America but only make it to our tables 1-2 times a year. Cranberries are delicious and full of beneficial antioxidants. This simple recipe is delicious and easy to prepare.

WHAT YOU'LL NEED...

- 3 cups of chopped apples
- 2 cups of fresh (or frozen) cranberries
- 1/3 cup of dried rose hips
- 1 tablespoon lemon juice
- 1 cup tart cherry juice
- 1 cup water
- 2 tablespoons ginger
- 1 teaspoon cinnamon
- 1/2 teaspoon nutmeg
- 1/4 teaspoon cloves
- Sugar or honey to taste
- Freshly whipped cream (optional)

To begin, place the fruits, lemon juice, apple cider and water into a pan and bring to a boil.

Reduce the heat so that it is on a low simmer. Continue to simmer for 20 minutes, stirring occasionally to prevent burning.

After twenty minutes the fruit should be soft and the mixture will look gelled or cooked down.

Add the spices and honey or sugar if desired. Stir for another two minutes.

This can be served immediately, although we find it's best after sitting for 24 hours. Serves 6-8 people.

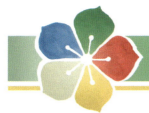

EXERCISE, BERRIES AND FRUIT

Rosehip Preserves

This is a yummy treat that I learned from someone who shared the recipe in the HerbMentor forums. She recommended using apple cider for the juice—I've come to love tart cherry juice. I'd recommend experimenting to see which you prefer.

WHAT YOU'LL NEED...

- de-seeded dried rose hips
- 1 teaspoon of honey (or to taste)
- 1 cinnamon stick
- tart cherry juice
- 8 ounce jar

Fill the 8 ounce jar a 1/4 of the way full with the rose hips.

Add the honey and cinnamon stick.

Fill the jar the rest of the way with the juice.

Let it sit overnight.

In the morning, the rosehips should have soaked up all the juice, leaving a pulpy preserve. Remove the cinnamon stick and use the spread on breads, scones, or ice cream.

Refrigerate and use quickly.

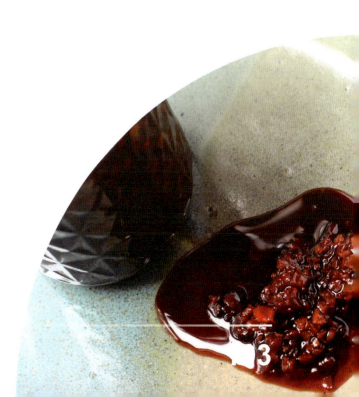

EXERCISE, BERRIES AND FRUIT

Rosehip Vinegar

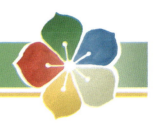

Rosehip vinegar is a sour and sweet preparation that makes a lovely salad dressing.

You can use fresh whole rosehips to make the vinegar or dried rosehips—both are delicious.

FOR FRESH ROSE HIPS:

WHAT YOU'LL NEED...

- whole fresh rosehips
- jar
- apple cider vinegar
- plastic lid

Fill a jar with the rose hips.

Then fill the jar with the vinegar.

Cover with a plastic lid.

Let sit for four weeks, shaking often.

When done, strain and use. Store in a cool dark place and use within six months.

FOR DRIED ROSE HIPS:

WHAT YOU'LL NEED...

- dried rose hips (either whole or de-seeded is fine)
- jar
- apple cider vinegar
- plastic lid

Fill the jar 1/3 to 1/2 way with the rose hips.

Then fill the jar with the vinegar.

Cover with a plastic lid.

Let sit for four weeks, shaking often.

When done, strain and use. Store in a cool dark place and use within a year.

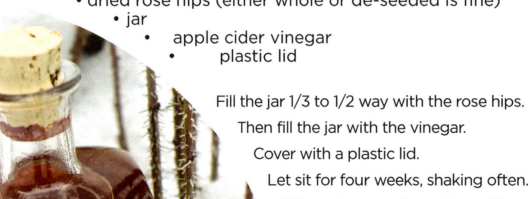

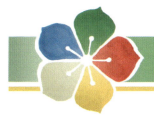

EXERCISE, BERRIES AND FRUIT

Sopa de Lima

This recipe is inspired by a traditional Yucatan (Mexico) soup that uses bitter oranges as the sour citrus kick. Since we don't often see these in the grocery stores up North, limes can be substituted instead.

My dad lives in the Yucatan, and this is his favorite soup—I can see why!

WHAT YOU'LL NEED...

- 8 corn tortillas
- 1/2 cup sunflower oil (or another oil for high heat cooking)
- salt to taste
- 2 tablespoons olive oil
- 1 medium onion, chopped
- 1 celery rib, thinly sliced
- 1 carrot, thinly sliced
- 1 jalapeño pepper, deseeded, and finely chopped
- 4 cloves garlic, minced
- 2 bay leaves
- 1 teaspoon dried oregano
- 1 teaspoon dried thyme
- 1 teaspoon freshly ground black pepper
- 1 large tomato, peeled, and chopped
- 8 cups bone broth or vegetable stock
- 1 & 1/2 pounds chicken cut into bite size pieces
- 2 green onions, finely chopped
- 1/3 cup freshly squeezed lime juice
- 1 lime sliced into wedges
- 1 large avocado, peeled, pitted, and coarsely chopped
- 2 tablespoons chopped fresh cilantro leaves

Cut the tortillas into 1/4-inch strips using a knife or pizza cutter. Heat the oil in a medium skillet. When the oil is very hot, fry the tortilla strips in small batches until lightly golden and crisp for 30 seconds to 1 minute. Transfer to a paper-towel-lined plate to drain. Season with salt to taste. Repeat until all tortilla strips have been fried.

In a large saucepan, heat the olive oil and sauté the onion, celery, and carrot. Continue to sauté until the vegetables have softened. Add the garlic, jalepeño, oregano, thyme, and black pepper

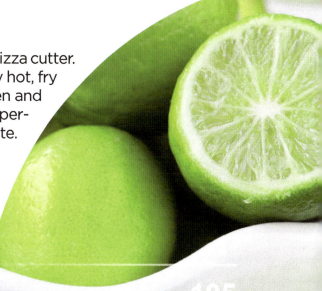

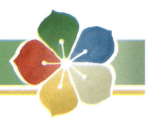

and cook another minute more. Add the tomato, soup stock, and chicken. Bring it to a boil. Reduce heat to a simmer and continue to cook until the chicken is cooked through (roughly 15 minutes).

Add the lime juice and green onions, and cook for another 3-5 minutes.

Serve into soup bowls. Garnish with the tortilla strips, avocado, a lime wedge, and cilantro.

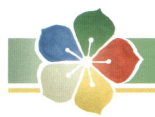

EXERCISE, BERRIES AND FRUIT

Spicy Lemonade

Lemonade made from fresh squeezed lemons is one of the best summer delights. This recipe warms up the traditional lemonade with spicy jalapeños and sage leaves.

This recipe is delicious as is. If you would like to serve it as a cocktail, add 1-2 shots of tequila or vodka to each glass.

WHAT YOU'LL NEED...

- 1 cup water
- 1/4 to 1/2 cup honey (depending on personal taste)
- 1/8 teaspoon salt
- 1 cup lemon juice (juice of about 6 large lemons), strained
- 1 jalapeño, cut into slices (remove seeds for a milder lemonade)
- 4 sprigs of sage
- 4 cups water

Place 1 cup of water, honey, and salt in a small saucepan. Gently heat the mixture, stirring just until the honey and water have fully combined. Remove from heat and let it cool.

Add the syrup mixture to the cup of lemon juice.

To prepare each glass...

Place one jalapeño slice (or more) and a sprig of fresh sage leaves in a glass. Muddle them well. (Muddling is a bartending term that basically means to bruise or mash fruits and herbs to release their flavor. I like to use a wooden spoon for this.)

Add 1 cup of the lemon syrup mixture and 1 cup of water. Add ice cubes, if desired and serve.

For a stronger jalapeño and sage flavor, combine all the ingredients in a large container several hours in advance before serving the individual glasses.

Makes up to 4 servings.

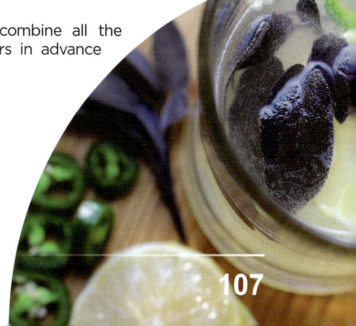

EXERCISE, FERMENTED FOODS

Strawberry Rhubarb Compote

This is a wonderful springtime treat. I adore rhubarb. While it's in season, I make lots of different compotes featuring this sour vegetable.

Compotes are essentially stewed fruits. You could also think of them as pie without the crust. They are easy to make. Also, they're gluten and dairy free.

If you don't have access to fresh tulsi, use mint instead.

WHAT YOU'LL NEED...

- 2 cups diced strawberries
- 1 cup diced rhubarb
- honey to taste
- two tablespoons of water
- 1/4 to 1/2 cup fresh tulsi leaves

Place the rhubarb and water in a small pan. Bring to a simmer. Keep simmering, stirring frequently, for about 7 minutes or until the rhubarb looks mushy.

Add the strawberries and honey. Stir for about a minute more until the strawberries are warmed and the honey is blended throughout.

Add the tulsi leaves, stir well, and remove from heat. Let it sit for 5 minutes and serve with freshly whipped cream, if desired.

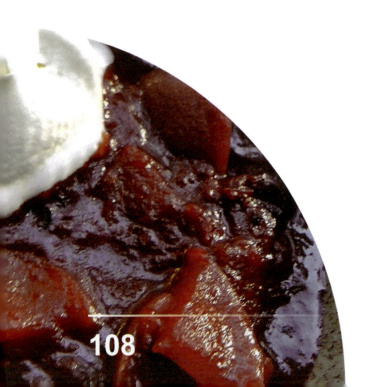

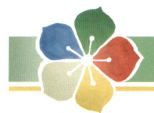

EXERCISE, FERMENTED FOODS

Beet Kvass

Beet kvass is a simple fermentation that uses beets, whey, and salt.

Beets are an amazing health food. They support liver health, they're high in antioxidants, and have been studied extensively for their ability to prevent chronic disease including cancer.

Fermenting beets to make this drink is a great way to get the benefits of live cultures as well as their beneficial qualities.

To make whey: Place 1 cup of live culture yogurt in a jelly bag suspended over a jar. The liquid that drips from the yogurt is whey. You can also use a couple tablespoons of live fermented sauerkraut juice.

For best results sterilize your equipment before starting.

WHAT YOU'LL NEED...

- 1/2 gallon jar
- beets chopped in 1/2 inch to fill the jar
- 2-3 tablespoons of whey
- 2 teaspoons sea salt
- water (best to use spring water rather than water that has been chlorinated)
- optional: orange zest, fennel seeds or some freshly chopped ginger

Place the chopped beets, whey, and salt into the 1/2 gallon jar. Add any optional spices as desired. Fill the jar with lukewarm spring water, leaving one inch head space at the top.

Cover it tightly with a lid.

Keep the jar at room temperature for 3-5 days. Open the jar every day. If scum appears on the top just spoon it off.

When it's done, the mixture will go from being a water consistency to a thicker consistency (kind of like tomato juice like V8). It will taste a bit salty and sour but mostly like thick beet juice.

Strain off the beets and store the beet kvass in the fridge. It will last about a week to a month.

I drink this about 4 ounces at a time.

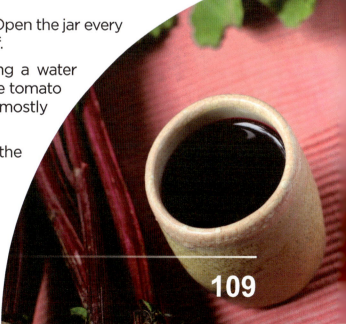

EXERCISE, FERMENTED FOODS

Fermented Veggies

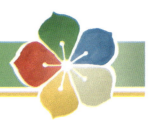

You can easily make your own fermented veggies. If you simply use cabbage this is commonly called sauerkraut (especially if you use caraway seeds for flavor), but there is no reason to stop with just cabbage!

My favorite veggie ferments also have carrots, Brussels sprouts, and garlic. You can use whatever variety of veggies in whatever quantity you like.

I recommend starting with a small batch, either one quart or a 1/2 gallon. For best results sterilize your equipment and wash your hands well before starting.

WHAT YOU'LL NEED...

- cabbage (I aim for 3/4 of the veggies being cabbage)
- carrots
- Brussels sprouts
- 2 cloves garlic, minced
- minced dried cayenne (optional for a spicier blend)
- 1 & 1/2 tablespoons kosher salt for 1/2 gallon of veggies
- 1/2 gallon wide mouth mason jar or fermenting crock
- small glass jar that fits inside the 1/2 gallon mason jar
- heavy stones to be used as weights

Begin by prepping your veggies. You'll want to cut the cabbage into thin ribbons and slice the carrots and Brussels sprouts fairly thin.

Mince the garlic.

Add the veggies to a large bowl in layers. Throw in a handful of veggies, sprinkle some of the salt. Use your hands to mash the veggies well. You can even use a thick wooden stick to pound the veggies. The goal is to coax them to break down and release their juices.

Keep adding the veggies and some salt. Continue with the mashing process.

When well mashed, place the veggies and salt mixture into the glass jar. Press it down firmly as you go to encourage more juices. Pour any juice from the bowl into the jar.

As you reach the top, leave enough space to place the small jar inside. Weigh it down with the stones. Cover the big jar with a plastic lid.

During the next 24 hours check on the fermented veggies frequently. Keep pressing the smaller jar down to encourage the juices to cover

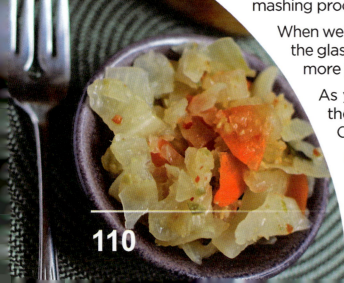

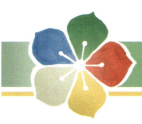

the veggies. After 24 hours, you want the juice to cover the veggies entirely. If this hasn't happened yet, add enough water to the jar to cover the veggies and another teaspoon of salt.

Storing your fermenting veggies at room temperature (65-75° F) is ideal. You should notice bubbles forming in the jar. Check on the veggies daily. If scum forms along the top just skim it off. Press the small jar down daily and make sure the liquid stays on the veggies.

The veggies will be done in 3-7 days. Keep tasting the mixture. When you like the taste, move it to the fridge. As long as the liquid is covering the veggies, they will last for a very long time.

EXERCISE, FERMENTED FOODS

Miso Soup

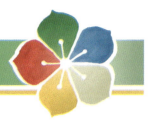

A simple miso soup is a wonderful start to a meal or can be an ideal meal for recovering from illness.

The salty taste has a soup with miso in it which has numerous ingredients, so this soup will be a simple broth that can easily be transformed into whatever soup suits your fancy.

I love making this simple broth with South River Miso. Their dandelion leek blend is my favorite, but all of them are fantastic. If you are new to miso, get their sampler pack. It's a good way to explore different kinds of miso. Of course, there are many different kinds of miso out there. Be sure to get it from the refrigerated section.

This incredibly simple recipe is made in minutes. You heat the liquid you want to use, remove from heat and add the miso. You don't want to cook the miso at high temperatures, as this will potentially kill the beneficial bacteria in the miso.

WHAT YOU'LL NEED...

- 8 ounces of water
- vegetable broth, or bone broth
- 1 teaspoon of miso

Heat the liquid until it simmers. Remove from heat and let it cool briefly.

Stir in the miso until it has mixed thoroughly. Enjoy.

Optional: Miso soup is often served with a bit of tofu and seaweed.

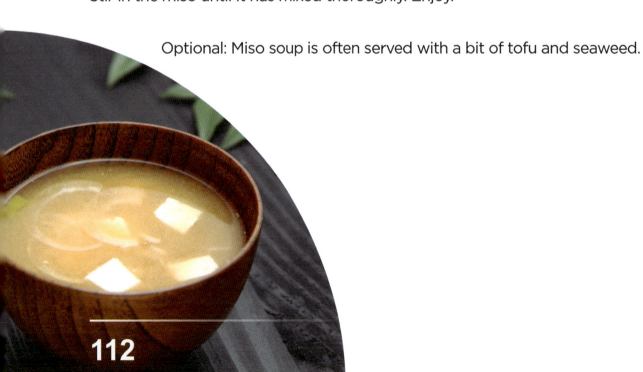

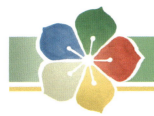

EXERCISE, FERMENTED FOODS

Yogurt

Making your own yogurt is incredibly simple. I like making my own yogurt because I can ensure I am using the best milk possible and avoid any unnecessary preservatives and sugars often found in commercial yogurt. Our local health food store carries raw milk from a small farm. If you don't have access to raw milk, be sure to get organic milk.

You can also make yogurt from goat milk or even coconut milk.

For best results, sterilize your stirring spoon, pot, thermometer, and glass jar with just-boiled water prior to starting.

WHAT YOU'LL NEED...

- 1/2 gallon milk
- yogurt starter (look for it in stores/online) OR 2-3 spoonfuls of yogurt with live cultures
- 1/2 gallon glass jar
- thermometer (with a range of 100° F to 185° F)
- a cooler and a towel

Begin by gently heating your milk. If you want to pasteurize your milk, heat it to 185° F. Stir frequently to avoid scalding it (or heat it in a double boiler).

Let this cool to 110° F. You can simply wait for it to cool on the counter, or you can put it in an ice bath to cool it down more quickly. Check it frequently to make sure it doesn't get too cool.

If you are using raw milk and want to keep it "raw" then only heat it to 110° degrees F. You will get more consistent results if you heat it to 185° F first. But I have made it plenty of times without heating it that high with great results.

When the milk has reached 110° F, add your yogurt culture or the spoonfuls of yogurt with live cultures. If using yogurt, it's imperative that it has live cultures in it.

Stir well. Pour the milk into a glass jar. Cover with a lid. Place into a cooler and wrap with a towel for increased insulation. Optional: You can put a hot water bottle in the cooler to warm it up a bit more. (You can also buy electric yogurt makers. I've never used them myself).

Let this sit without moving it for 8 hours. I put mine in overnight. By morning it should thicken into a yogurt. Store in the fridge. It will last for a week or longer.

Enjoy your homemade yogurt. Use fruit to make smoothies with it or try a savory tzatziki sauce.

BITTER

Ayurveda Elements

Ether and Wind
cold, dry and light

TCM Organs

Heart and Small Intestines
yin

Chemical constituents

glycosides, alkaloids

How we use the bitter taste

Bitter tastes are cooling and drying. When the tongue detects bitterness it increases salivary secretions, which creates a cascade of digestive secretions from HCL to bile to pancreatic enzymes; thus, it promotes digestion.

Examples

Dandelion leaves, kale, oregon grape root, and gentian.

Contraindications

Coldness, debility

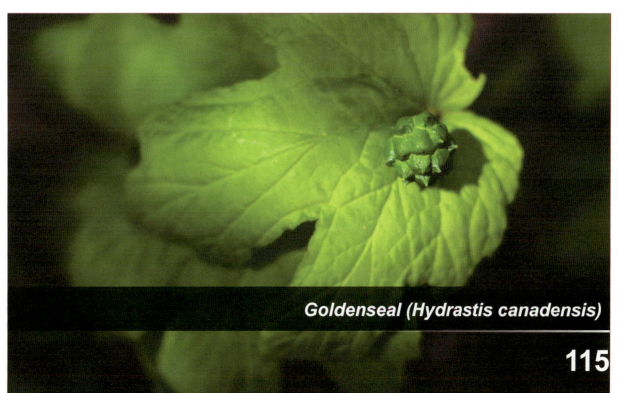

Goldenseal (Hydrastis canadensis)

EXERCISE, INTRODUCTION
Bitterness Scale

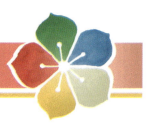

Try herbs in these three categories to develop an understanding of the different levels of bitterness within the bitter materia medica.

MILD

Dandelion root
Brussels Sprouts
Coffee

MODERATE

Dandelion leaf (young)
Artichoke Leaf
Hops

SUPER BITTER

Boneset
Gentian
Andrographis

AROMATIC BITTERS

One subcategory of bitters are the aromatic bitters. These herbs are both pungent or aromatic as well as strongly bitter. They tend to be more warming in nature.

    Elecampane
        Turmeric
            Chamomile

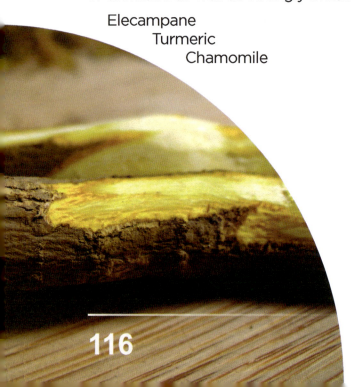

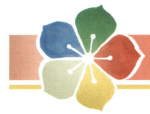

EXERCISE, ALTERATIVES AND LYMPHAGOGUES

Alterative Blend

This is a basic alterative blend that is generally safe for most people. It is especially suited to supporting liver health and moving lymphatic congestion.

WHAT YOU'LL NEED...

- 40 milliliters dandelion root tincture
- 40 milliliters burdock root tincture
- 20 milliliters red root tincture
- 15 milliliters fresh cleavers tincture
- 5 milliliters fennel seed tincture

Combine these tinctures together in a 4 ounce dropper bottle. This can be taken at 60-90 drops three to five times a day.

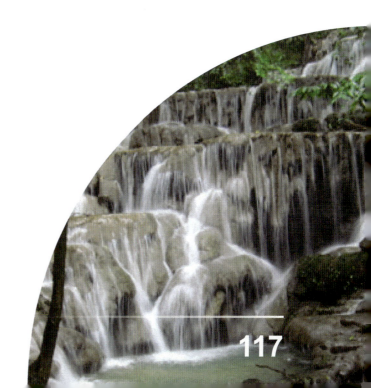

EXERCISE, ALTERATIVES AND LYMPHAGOGUES

Marinated Burdock Root

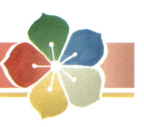

Burdock root is a beloved, nutritious herb with gentle but alterative actions. It is commonly eaten in stew pots or in stir fries.

We almost always have a jar of this wonderful recipe around. It makes a great garnish and a fancy hors d'oeuvre. I learned this recipe with Karen Sherwood, and I believe she learned it from herbalist Eaglesong at Ravencroft Gardens.

WHAT YOU'LL NEED...

- 6-8 burdock roots
- 2 cups of water
- 2 cups of Tamari or soy sauce
- 2 cups of balsamic vinegar
- 4 cloves of garlic
- 1 piece of ginger

Wash and thinly slice the burdock roots.

Slice the garlic and ginger into matchstick size pieces.

Add the burdock root, garlic, and ginger to a medium skillet with the 2 cups of water.

Sauté until the burdock becomes tender.

Add Tamari and vinegar. Bring the temperature of the mixture up to simmering.

Store in the refrigerator. It keeps for many months.

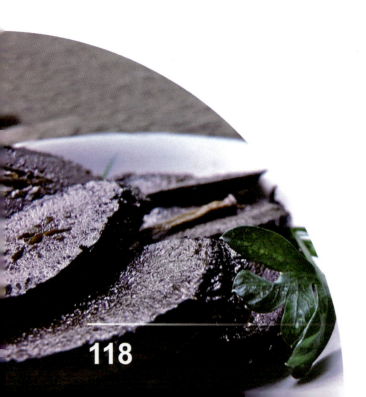

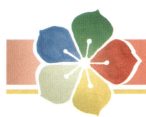

EXERCISE, ALTERATIVES AND LYMPHAGOGUES

Rich Roasted Reishi Tea

This is one of my favorite tea blends. It combines the rich roasted flavor of the chicory and dandelion with the immunosupportive adaptogen qualities of reishi mushroom.

The blend has numerous benefits, but it's especially supportive to liver health.

WHAT YOU'LL NEED...

- 10 grams roasted dandelion root
- 7 grams roasted chicory root
- 6 grams reishi mushroom
- 12 ounces of water

Simmer the roots and reishi for 45 minutes to an hour.

Strain. Add milk and/or honey, if desired. I love to sip this while eating another one of my favorite bitter tonics such as dark chocolate.

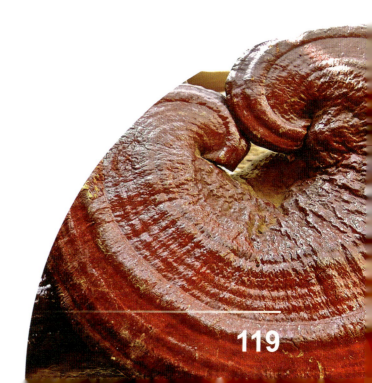

EXERCISE, INTRODUCTION

Dandelion Tea

Roasted dandelion root tea is one of my favorite beverages. It's warm and rich, slightly nutty and bitter in flavor. Many people call it a "coffee substitute".

I like it with cream and piping hot in the winter. During the summer months, I'll take it chilled after spending days in the hot sun.

You can order roasted dandelion roots from Mountain Rose Herbs (or possibly find them in your local herb store). You can also harvest your own roots or buy them unroasted then roast them yourself.

To do this, I place the dried cut root in a dry cast iron pan on medium heat. I stir frequently and consider them roasted when the root has darkened in color and when there is a rich smell emanating from the roots. Once they are cooled, I store them in a covered container for convenient use.

WHAT YOU'LL NEED...

- 1 heaping tablespoon of roasted dandelion root
- 8 ounces of water

Simmer the root in the water for 10-20 minutes. You'll get more beneficial properties if you have the patience to wait for 20 minutes, but it will taste fine after 10.

Once it is done, strain, add honey and/or milk to taste.

Roasted dandelion tea makes a great base for chai recipes.

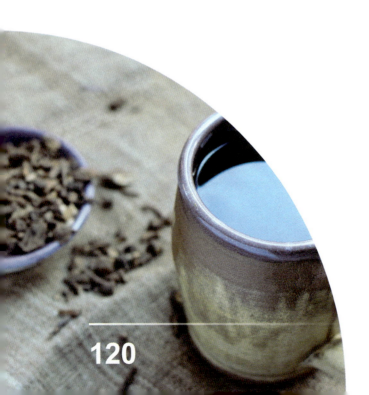

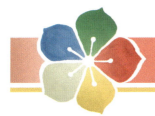

EXERCISE, BALANCE BLOOD SUGAR

Bitter Melon Juice

Bitter melon is famous for its bitterness and known for lowering blood sugar.

That hasn't kept people from eating it though. It's a common vegetable in Asian cuisine. You can find bitter melons in Asian grocery stores, both fresh and frozen.

When I recommend bitter melon for reducing blood sugar levels (alongside diet, exercise and lifestyle changes), I suggest people take it as a fresh juice. In order to do this on a regular basis, you'll need to have access to it fresh. I hear it's easy to grow in temperate climates.

WHAT YOU'LL NEED...

- several fresh bitter melons
- juicer

Juice the fresh bitter melons until you have 1-3 ounces of juice. This will be bitter. You can mix it with other freshly juiced vegetables that have a milder flavor or simply drink it down in one shot.

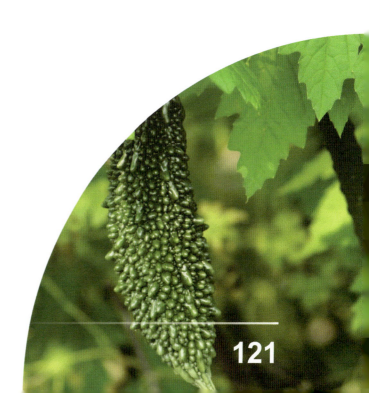

EXERCISE, BALANCE BLOOD SUGAR

Spiced Coffee

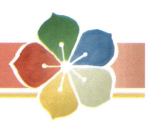

Coffee is so vilified that it can be surprising to learn that it has many health benefits. It's high in antioxidants, has many qualities found in the bitter taste, and can help lower blood sugar levels.

This delicious spiced coffee blend contains cinnamon and cardamom. Both help to stimulate digestion. Cinnamon is well known for its blood sugar regulating effects.

WHAT YOU'LL NEED...

- 15 grams of coffee (or however much you regularly use for one cup of coffee)
- 1 teaspoon cinnamon powder
- 1/2 teaspoon cardamom

I use a melitta to brew my coffee. I place all the ingredients in the melitta and pour enough hot water for my cup of coffee.

This recipe can easily be used in any number of coffee brewing devices.

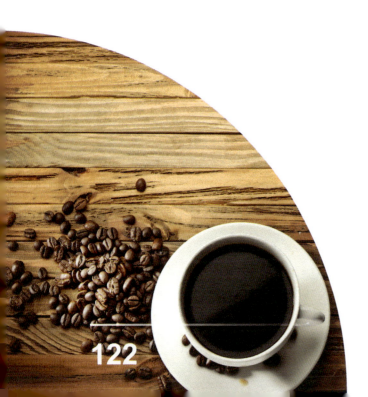

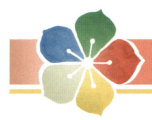

EXERCISE, LAXATIVE

Rooty Laxative

This gentle laxative blend comes from herbalist Rosemary Gladstar. All three of these roots gently promote bowel movement. Yellow dock and dandelion are both bitter alteratives, while licorice is a decidedly sweet demulcent.

If you have high blood pressure, omit the licorice and substitute flax seeds.

WHAT YOU'LL NEED...

- 10 grams of dandelion root
- 7 grams of yellow dock root
- 1-2 grams of licorice root
- 1 pint of water

Simmer the roots in the water for 20-30 minutes. Strain.

Drink throughout the day. You should see results within 12 hours.

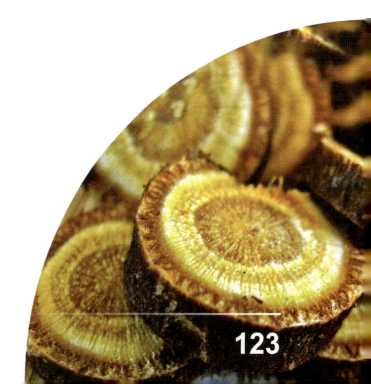

EXERCISE, LAXATIVE

Triphala

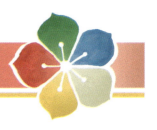

Triphala is probably the most famous and most used of Ayurvedic formulas.

Triphala is a blend of three fruits.

Amalaki *(Emblica officinalis)*
Bibhitaki *(Terminalia belerica)*
Haritaki *(Terminalia chebula)*

Triphala is both nourishing and detoxifying. It gently supports regular bowel movements. In addition, it supports liver function while also providing adaptogenic properties. It's my most used herbal formulation for constipation.

How to best take Triphala?

I generally recommend 1-6 grams of triphala taken at night.

Triphala is commonly taken as a powder stirred into hot water.

To make this tea, start with a 1/2 teaspoon of the powder in a cup. Stir in 8 ounces of hot water. Drink. You may need to add additional water to the cup to ensure you get most of the powder.

After a few days of trying 1/2 teaspoon, slowly raise your triphala amount by half teaspoon amounts.

The idea is to get as much triphala in as possible without creating loose stools.

If you take 1 teaspoon and have a firm bowel movement the next day, great! If you take 1 & 1/2 teaspoons the next night and have loose stools the next morning, go back to the one teaspoon.

If you can't tolerate the taste of the powder, encapsulate the powder or buy tablets.

Like the tea, start with a low dose and slowly increase to bowel intolerance.

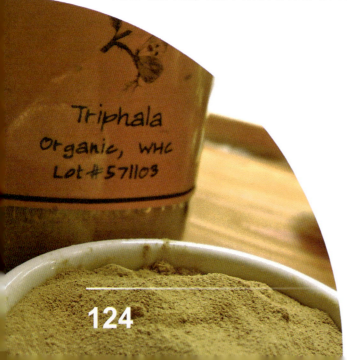

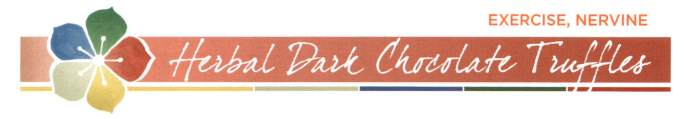

EXERCISE, NERVINE

Herbal Dark Chocolate Truffles

Chocolate truffles are so alluring. The earthy and bitter taste of chocolate is combined with a perfect melting sensation.

Most of the truffles you buy in the store really are junk food. They have strange preservatives and colorings, tons of sugar, a minimal amount of actual cacao content, and lots of milk (which further decreases the benefits of cacao).

This truffle blend is high in cacao, has minimal amounts of sugars (in the form of honey), and uses coconut milk instead of dairy.

I hope you love these as much as we do! We often give them as gifts during the holidays and get rave reviews.

WHAT YOU'LL NEED...

- 8 ounces of dark chocolate (I use 4 ounces of 100% cacao and 4 ounces of bittersweet chocolate)
- 2/3 cup coconut milk
- 2 teaspoons vanilla extract
- 1 teaspoon powdered cinnamon
- 1/2 teaspoon powdered nutmeg
- powdered cacao and powdered roses for rolling

Begin by chopping or pounding the chocolate into pea size pieces. Place this into a medium sized bowl along with the vanilla, powdered cinnamon, and nutmeg.

Warm the coconut milk slowly before it starts to simmer. Pour this immediately into the bowl with chocolate.

Let this stand for one minute and stir with a whisk until the chocolate is melted and has a smooth consistency.

Note: Most of the time, this process works great when I make these. One or two times, I didn't make the chocolate pieces small enough and it didn't fully melt with the coconut milk. When this happened I placed the chocolate in a double boiler and heated it slowly until the chocolate melted.

Once you have the truffle sauce, it needs to cool to a semi-hard consistency. I don't have a foolproof method for this. I suggest keeping it in the fridge or freezer and checking it frequently. It needs to be soft enough to form into a ball, yet hard enough to roll without falling apart.

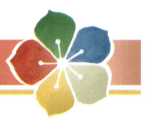

Once the desired consistency is reached you can start rolling. Scoop the mixture into bite sized pieces. Using clean hands, roll it into a ball.

Once they are all rolled, I suggest rolling them in a powder. I think it's nice to have a variety of powders within a single batch. I suggest playing around with the following…

- cacao powder
- cacao powder mixed with cinnamon
- cacao powder mixed with powdered rose petals
- powdered rose petals

Variations

Many powdered herbs can be used in this recipe. Ginger, cayenne, and rose are just a few ideas.

Orange zest can be added to the truffles themselves or even used to roll the truffles in.

Coconut can be used to roll the truffles in.

Baking extracts come in all sorts of flavors and can be added here (mint, coffee, orange, etc).

You can infuse a variety of herbs into the warmed coconut milk to impart different flavors.

Earl Grey: Heat the coconut milk and add a few teabags of earl grey. Let it sit for 5 minutes, remove tea bags, heat the cream again, and proceed as normal. You may need to add a bit more coconut to this.

Lavender: Add 2 teaspoons of lavender to the warmed coconut milk. Let it sit 5 minutes, strain off the lavender, reheat, and proceed.

As you can see this is just the beginning of finding your own favorite truffle recipe.

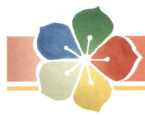

EXERCISE, NERVINE

Chocolate Mousse Cake

The following recipe is a delicious pairing of cardamom and cacao. To make this recipe, you begin by making chocolate from cacao butter and cacao powder. This ensures you've got really dark and rich chocolate with all of those healthy benefits.

We've made this recipe countless times in the past year and have taken it to many potlucks and dinner gatherings. Each time we have a list of people who desperately want the recipe.

WHAT YOU'LL NEED...

- 130 grams of cacao butter
- 90 grams of sifted cacao powder (plus a bit more for decoration)
- 4 tablespoons of honey (or to taste)
- a 13.5 ounce can of coconut milk
- 1 tablespoon of cardamom
- 2 eggs
- sliced almonds (optional)

Over a double boiler, melt the cacao butter.

Remove from the heat and add the cacao powder. Mix well.

Add the honey, coconut milk, cardamom, and eggs. Mix well.

Pour into a slightly oiled pie pan. (I use coconut oil.)

Cook at 350° for 30 minutes.

When it's done, the top should be cracked, but the middle should still be soft and wiggly.

Cool overnight to allow it to set. Sprinkle with sliced almonds, if desired.

Sprinkle some cocoa powder on top before serving.

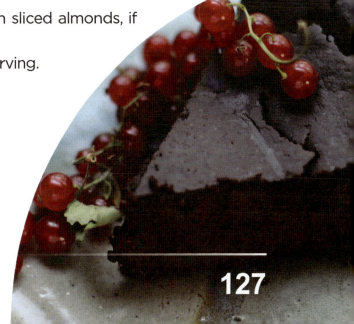

EXERCISE, NERVINE

Relaxing Nervines

In the pungent taste, we explored pungent relaxing nervines. Now that we are being introduced to bitter relaxing nervines, you might try experimenting with them to see which ones you have a special affinity for.

Sometimes it isn't an either/or situation. Try combining the bitter relaxing nervines with pungent relaxing nervines, too.

Here's a listing of herbs to choose from. These work well as teas or tinctures.

In this exercise, we aren't just developing our sense of taste, but we're paying close attention to how the herbs make us feel.

Bitter Relaxing Nervines	Pungent Relaxing Nervines
California Poppy *Eschscholzia californica*	Chamomile* *Matricaria recutita*
Hops *Humulus lupulus*	Lavender* *Lavandula spp.*
Motherwort *Leonurus cardiaca*	Lemon Balm *Melissa officinalis*
Passion flower *Passiflora incarnata*	Nutmeg *Myristica fragrans*
Skullcap *Scutellaria lateriflora*	Sage *Salvia officinalis*
Vervain *Verbena hastata*	Tulsi *Ocimum sanctum*
Vervain *Verbena officinalis*	Valerian *Valeriana officinalis*
Wild Lettuce *Latuca spp*	Kava *Piper methysticum*

*these herbs are aromatic and bitter and tend to be warming

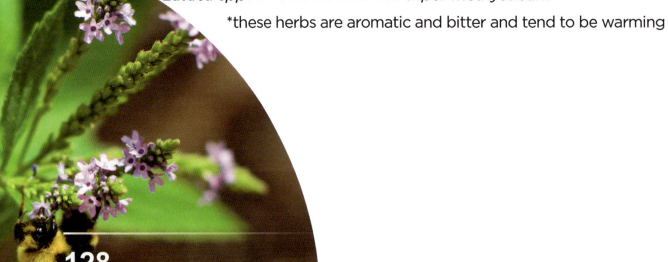

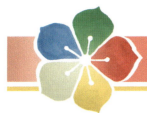

EXERCISE, ALTERATIVES AND LYMPHAGOGUES

Skullcap Tea

Skullcap (*Scutellaria lateriflora*) is the perfect example of a bitter relaxing nervine. Called "blisswort" by Kiva Rose, this sweet little plant can relieve anxiety and promote sleep. It's frequently used as a tincture. I love to take it as a strong tea to promote sleep.

In this recipe, I use a lot of skullcap in a small amount of water. I've found the less I drink just before bed the better.

WHAT YOU'LL NEED...

- 5 grams skullcap leaf
- 8 ounces of water

Steep the skullcap in just-boiled water, covered, for 10-20 minutes. Strain.

Drink about an hour before bed.

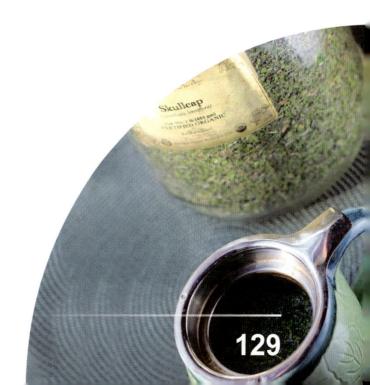

EXERCISE, NERVINE

Sleep Blend

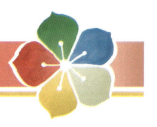

This all-purpose sleep blend has helped many people find their zzz's at night. You'll see that this blend includes mostly cooling, bitter relaxing nervines. If someone has more signs of coldness, I will substitute valerian for California poppy.

This blend has mild pain relieving abilities and can help if pain is preventing someone from sleeping.

This can be taken in smaller doses during the day to help relieve stress and anxiety, also.

WHAT YOU'LL NEED...
equal parts tincture of...

- California Poppy *(Eschscholzia californica)*
- Hops *(Humulus lupulus)*
- Skullcap leaves *(Scutellaria laterifolia)*
- Chamomile *(Matricaria recutita)*

Mix the four herbal tinctures into your desired container and keep it by your bed for easy use.

Tips for taking the tincture

Start with 30-60 drops, 30 minutes before bed, and then another 30-60 drops right before bed.

If you're still awake 20 minutes after going to bed, try another 30-60 drops. Keep titrating the dose every ten minutes until you fall asleep.

Over time you should get a good feel for how much you need to take for a good night's rest.

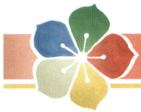

EXERCISE, RELAXING DIAPHORETIC

Boneset Tea

There's an interesting thing about boneset tea—if you drink it while you're healthy, you'll probably hate it. It's disastrously and amazingly bitter. Even if you think you love bitters, you will most likely detest this.

However, if you sip boneset tea while you're feverish and your body is full of the aches and pains of the fever process, you'll probably come to adore this tea and the amazing relief that it brings. I've heard several people say it tastes entirely different while sick. Still bitter but much more pleasant.

Because boneset is so very bitter, if you drink too much of it too quickly, it can make you nauseous or even vomit. I suggest drinking the warm tea in frequent but small sips while you have a fever with aches and pains. I generally recommend it. It could be blended with other relaxing diaphoretic herbs like elderflowers.

WHAT YOU'LL NEED...

- 10 grams of boneset leaf *(Eupatorium perfoliatum)*
- 1 pint of just-boiled water

Steep the boneset in the water for 10-20 minutes. Strain.

Drink in small frequent sips.

Decrease the frequency of your sips if you feel queasy at all.

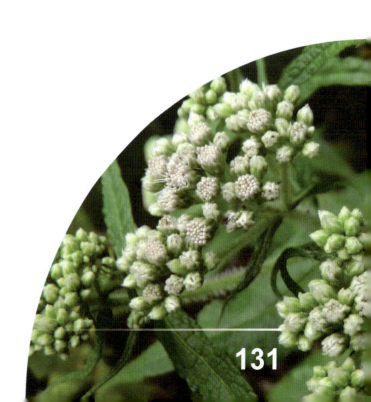

EXERCISE, RELAXING DIAPHORETIC

Elderflower Tea

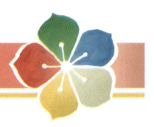

This is a very old western recipe that is considered a general formula for colds and the flu. I've given it to countless people and seen it relieve a lot of discomfort associated with these illnesses. It's quite effective, but gentle enough for most people and even children.

Both elderflowers and yarrow are used as relaxing diaphoretics, making this blend especially well suited for people with fevers who feel hot and are restless.

This may have been one of the first herbal formulas I ever learned. I love its simplicity, and that many of these plants grow right outside my door. Most traditional formulas only include the first three ingredients, but I think the rose hips make a nice addition.

Peppermint, spearmint or even bee balm *(Monarda fistulosa)* are wonderful mints to use in this blend.

WHAT YOU'LL NEED...

- 1 part elderflower
- 1 part yarrow
- 1/2 part mint
- 1/2 part rose hips

I like to have a large batch of this already mixed up.

To make the tea I steep a 1/2 cup of the mixture in one pint of water for thirty minutes. Strain and then sip while warm.

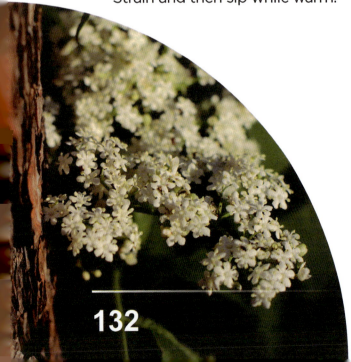

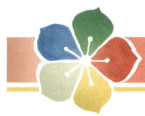

EXERCISE, STIMULATES DIGESTION, BITTERS

Creamy Greens Soup

Here is a creamed green soup. I suggest using a mixture of greens, including beet greens, collard greens, kale and at least a cup of dandelion leaf greens. The kale, beet greens and collards are exceptionally nutritious while the bitterness of the dandelions brings the soup to life.

WHAT YOU'LL NEED...

- 3 cups homemade chicken stock
- 6-7 cups of chopped veggies
- salt and freshly ground pepper to taste

Bring the stock to a simmer and add the greens and salt and pepper. Simmer for a couple minutes or until the greens are just tender.

Using an immersion blender, puree the soup. (Or let cool and use a blender or food processor.)

This soup can be dazzled up using some pungent spices like garlic, onions or herbs.

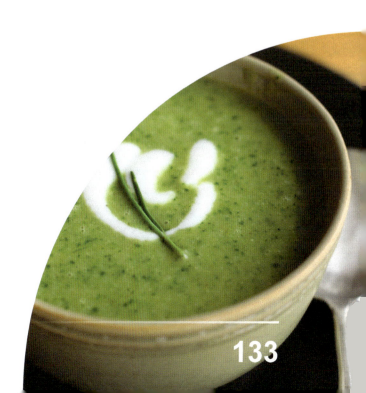

EXERCISE, STIMULATES DIGESTION, BITTERS

Dandelion Pesto

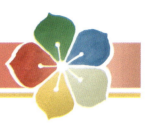

I love this pesto as a dip, on bread, pasta, salmon, or even a couple tablespoons on eggs.

Use fresh young dandelion leaves for this recipe. If you don't have an area to harvest these near you, ask your local grocery store if they can order dandelion leaves.

WHAT YOU'LL NEED...

- 2-4 crushed cloves of garlic
- 1/2 cup cold pressed olive oil
- 2-3 cups of young dandelion leaves
- 1/4 cup of freshly grated parmesan cheese
- a dash of sea salt
- a squirt of lemon juice (optional)
- 1/4 cup of ground nuts (walnuts, pine nuts)

I prefer to make this type of mixture in a food processor. If you have one of these handy devices, simply place all the ingredients in the processor and blend until well mixed together.

If you do not have a food processor, you can make this in a blender. Since I've burned out many blenders doing this, here are my very precise instructions on how to make dandelion pesto and not break your blender in the process.

- Place oil, garlic, and salt in the blender along with half of the dandelion leaves.
- Blend well and add the other half of the leaves. When finished blending, it should be of a good consistency although still a little runny.
    - If you have a strong blender, add the rest of the ingredients and blend. If not, pour the mixture into a bowl and add desired amounts of parmesan cheese, ground nuts, and lemon juice.

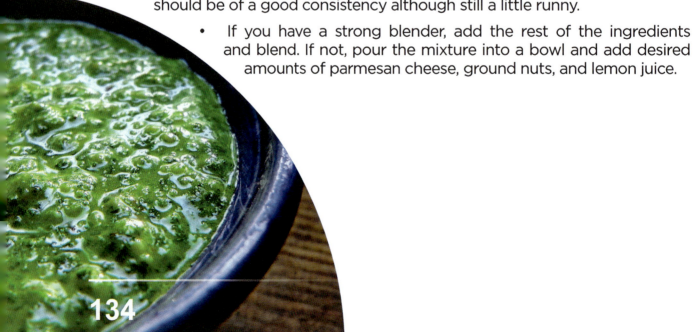

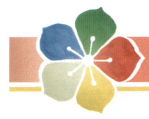

EXERCISE, STIMULATES DIGESTION, BITTERS

Make your own bitters

If you are an herbal nerd, creating your own bitter extracts is really fun. There are so many possibilities for your own unique bitter blend. Be sure to keep track of what you do so you can replicate your soon-to-be amazing creations.

Bitters are all the rage right now, and I've even seen herbalists host bitter "parties" where a group of herbalists send out their unique bitter blends to everyone in the "party".

If you really want to get into bitter blends, then I highly recommend the book _Bitters: A Spirited History of a Classic Cure-All, with Cocktails, Recipes, and Formulas_ by Brad Thomas. Not only does it recount the interesting history of bitters, but it also includes some really interesting bitter recipes.

For those of you who are wild crafters or gardeners, one way to make your bitter blend especially unique is to use herbs only harvested or grown by you.

Bitter blends are essential to bitter tincture formulas (alcohol extract). When making bitter blends, I like to use brandy or 50% vodka as the menstruum.

When you first start making bitters, you may want to tincture individual herbs and blend them into a finished product. This allows you to experiment with smaller amounts. Once you get the hang of how to make delicious bitter blends you can start combining all the herbs and spices into one jar (like the pear spiced bitters blend).

These bitter herbal extracts can be used in mixed drinks or simply taken in small quantities (5-15 drops) before meals to promote digestion.

Here are the basic components of making your own bitters.

Bitter Herbs

Of course, your bitter blends is going to include some bitters! Experiment with how bitter you would like it. Generally bitters have a distinct bitter taste, but some bitters have a pleasant taste.

Tip: I like adding dandelion root and elecampane root to my bitter blends. These roots can be high in inulin, which is a pre-biotic. Think of it as a healthy food for your gut flora promoting digestive health. If you make your own tinctures of dandelion root and/or elecampane, the milky residue at the bottom of the jar is the inulin. Be sure not to strain it out! If you buy dandelion root tincture or elecampane root, the inulin may be missing as it's frequently strained out to give the end product a clear consistency.

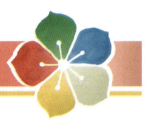

Other bitter herbs that are frequently used in blends include artichoke leaf, gentian root, and dandelion leaf. Practically any herbal bitter can be used.

Tasty Carminative Spices

These spices can "warm up" the bitters blend and give it a more nuanced and enjoyable flavor. Many bitter blends include angelica (an aromatic bitter) and spices like ginger, cloves, fennel, cardamom, etc.

Perhaps a Touch of Sweetness

Adding a sweet component to your blends isn't necessary, but it can add a deeper complexity to the overall taste. This can be as simple as adding a touch of honey to the mix or by incorporating fresh or dried fruit.

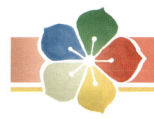

EXERCISE, STIMULATES DIGESTION, BITTERS

Roasted Radicchio

Having bitters with meals doesn't have to include alcohol extracts or specially prepared teas, it can simply be the natural bitter taste in your food. Thanks to herbalist and bitter aficionado Jim McDonald for this recipe.

WHAT YOU'LL NEED...

meat
- 1-2 pounds chicken breast (brined and marinated in balsamic vinegar and olive oil, with a bit of salt, pepper, and garlic powder)

plants
- 2 heads radicchio
- (ideally fresh) thyme
- garlic (slivered or powder)
- toasted sesame seeds

lipids/cheeses
- olive oil

stuff in bottles
- awesome tasting balsamic vinegar, or a balsamic reduction

1. Pre-heat oven to 400° F.
2. Quarter a head of radicchio. Drizzle with olive oil and sprinkle over with sea salt, pepper, slivered garlic or a bit of garlic powder, and thyme.
3. Roast for 12 minutes. Turn and continue for another 6-8 minutes.
4. While your radicchio is roasting, grill up your chicken.
5. Remove the radicchio. Cut the radicchio and the chicken up into bite sized pieces. Combine and toss together. I usually add some more fresh thyme and sesame seeds.
6. Drizzle a good balsamic vinegar to taste. If you don't have balsamic that's so good you'd lick spills up off the floor, you can concentrate the flavor by making a reduction. Put your balsamic in a pot and reduce till thick and syrupy. The flavor should be bold and sweet.

This recipe is crazy awesome with medium rare venison backstraps. You can also grill up portabellas or shiitakes instead of using chicken. But the bitterness of the radicchio is the star of this recipe. I like making it simple without much else added so I can savor that.

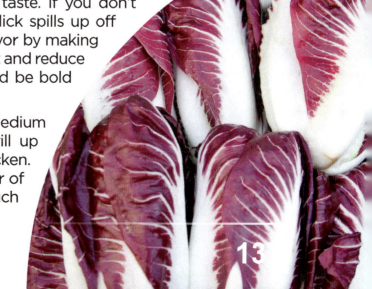

EXERCISE, VERMICIDE
Parasite Formula

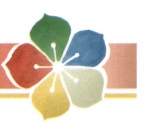

This formula is based on the work of Hannah Krueger. As I mentioned in the vermicide video, parasites are best addressed with vermicide herbs as well as the appropriate diet and eliminating therapies.

These herbs are generally safe but can be potentially harsh on the digestive system, causing nausea or other abdominal discomfort. While taking vermicide herbs, avoid eating sugar or excessive carbs. Take a gentle laxative to make sure the bowels are moving well.

WHAT YOU'LL NEED...

- wormwood powder *(Artemisia absinthium)*
- green black walnut hull powder *(Juglans nigra)*
- quassia powder *(Quassia amara)*
- cloves powder *(Syzygium aromaticum)*

Combine the powdered herbs in equal parts. Take 1/2 gram to 6 grams throughout the day.

You can mix the powder into hot water, but this will taste awful. You may want to encapsulate it.

Herbalist Phyllis Light recommends taking vermicide herbs during the full moon since parasites tend to be more active during this time. Depending on the particular parasite, it may take days, weeks, or even months to fully resolve.

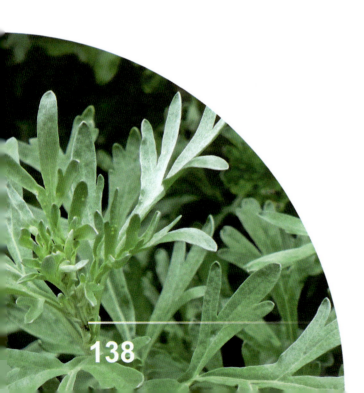

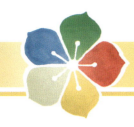

SWEET

Ayurveda Elements

Earth and Water
wet, cold and heavy

TCM Organs

Spleen and Stomach
yang

Chemical constituents

Sugars, fats, proteins, carbs, polysaccharides, and GAGs

How we use the sweet tast

The sweet taste is considered building and strengthening. It can moisten tissues, soothe inflammation, and nourish the blood. It can relieve burning sensations (think of reaching for milk after eating hot peppers) and promote calmness and centeredness.

Examples

The sweet taste is found in milk, honey, sugars, grains, sweet vegetables (root vegetables), meats, and fish. Sweet-tasting herbs include marshmallow, slippery elm, and astragalus root.

Contraindications

Respiratory congestion, diabetes, fever, weak digestion, feelings of heaviness, lethargy and parasites.

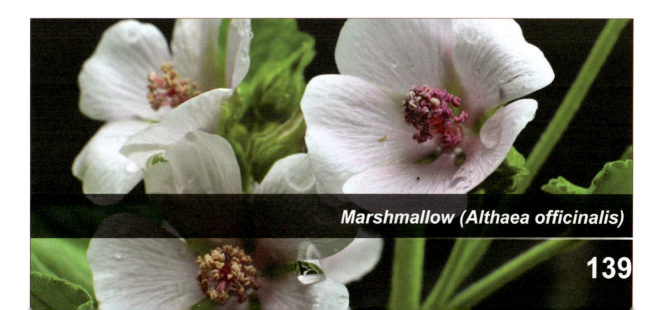

Marshmallow (Althaea officinalis)

EXERCISE, INTRODUCTION

Tasting Sweet Herbs

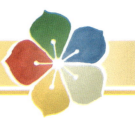

In the introductory video to this course, I explained that sometimes herbs are classified as having a certain taste even though it may not have that overt taste.

When we think of sweet, most of us immediately think of the sweetness of sugar or honey. Sweet herbs are rarely that sweet.

In fact, some of them aren't all that sweet at all! Ginseng, ashwaganda, and many medicinal mushrooms are classified as being sweet because they are building and nourishing, not because they taste like candy.

In this exercise, you'll be tasting some "sweet" herbs to get a better understanding of the sweet taste in herbal medicine. Over time, you'll probably be able to taste those elusive sweet tastes in these less sweet herbs.

You can taste these herbs using any preparation, but I recommend tasting the powder or making a tea to have the more pure taste test.

Licorice *(Glycyrrhiza glabra)*

Stevia *(Stevia spp.)*

Marshmallow root *(Althaea officinalis)*

Astragalus *(Astragalus membranaceous)*

Ginseng *(Panax ginseng)*

Ashwaganda *(Withania somnifera)*

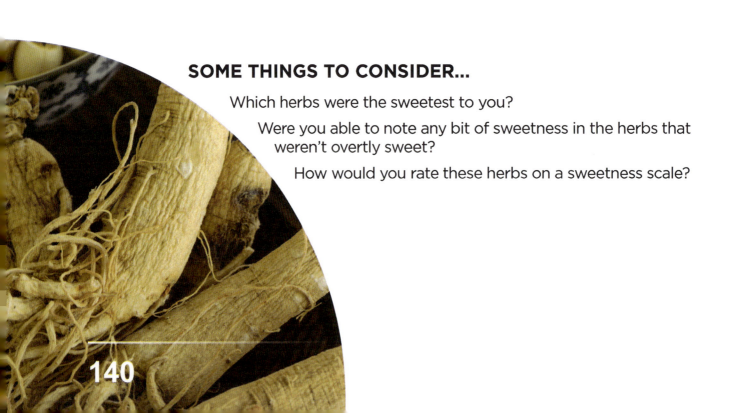

SOME THINGS TO CONSIDER...

Which herbs were the sweetest to you?

Were you able to note any bit of sweetness in the herbs that weren't overtly sweet?

How would you rate these herbs on a sweetness scale?

Marshmallows

You'll often read that the marshmallow plant *(Althaea officinalis)* was once used to make marshmallows. That's right! Those spongy and sweet treats that are an essential ingredient to S'mores and hot chocolate had their roots in the herbal world!

For the past few weeks I've been trying to dig up those recipes and create my own version. I wanted to create something original, so I added some color and rose hydrosol. Doesn't chocolate rose S'mores sound elegant?! Maybe we can market them as marshmallows with a grown up taste.

WHAT YOU'LL NEED...

- 1/2 cup rose hydrosol
- 1/2 cup water
- 1 tablespoon marshmallow root powder
- 1-2 tablespoons of hibiscus flowers (these make the marshmallows pink!)
- 1 cup honey
- 2 tablespoons plus 1 teaspoon unflavored gelatin
- 1 teaspoon vanilla extract
- pinch of salt

OTHER...

- hand mixer
- 8x8 pan
- candy Thermometer
- sauce Pan

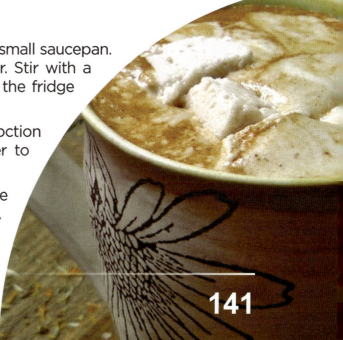

Bring the water and rose hydrosol to a boil in a small saucepan. Add the marshmallow root and hibiscus flower. Stir with a whisk. Simmer for five minutes and place it in the fridge until it cools.

Strain the marshmallow and hibiscus decoction through a fine mesh sieve. Add enough water to equal a full cup.

Take half of the marshmallow mixture and place it in a medium-sized bowl and add gelatin to it. Set it aside.

Take the other half of the mixture in a small

EXERCISE, INTRODUCTION

Marshmallows

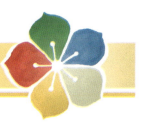

saucepan along with the honey, vanilla extract and the salt.

Bring to a simmer. Place the candy thermometer in the mixture until it reaches 240° (soft ball) then remove from heat.

Using a hand mixer begin to mix the marshmallow and gelatin mixture on low. Slowly add the hot marshmallow and honey mixture while continuing to mix.

Once the two mixtures have been combined continue to whip on high for another 5-10 minutes.

Pour the mixture onto an 8x8 pan lined with natural parchment paper that has been oiled.

Let these sit for a few hours until they are set up and firm.

Slice it with a knife. These are a little sticky. You could roll them in rose petal powder or powdered sugar if you wanted them less sticky.

Enjoy these marshmallows any way you would enjoy the store-bought variety. I decided to go above and beyond for you all and force myself to try them in my hot cocoa. It was incredible!

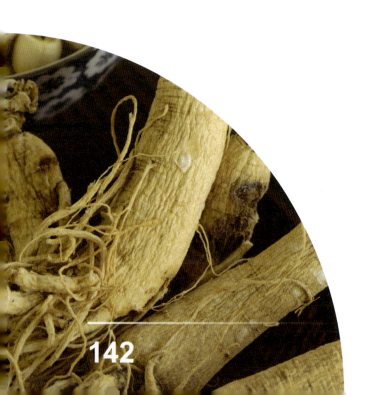

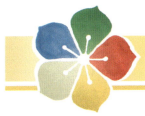

EXERCISE, INTRODUCTION
Vanilla Extract

Vanilla may be one of the most popular dessert flavors. From straight up vanilla ice cream to baked goods made with vanilla extract, most of us have been tasting vanilla all our lives.

Vanilla is one of the most expensive spices on the market. Buying the pure extract is costly. If you're not careful about the quality of the extract you're buying, you could be consuming petrochemicals and by-products from the wood industry. Yuck!

Before we learn how to make our own vanilla extract, here's some interesting historical information about vanilla.

The vanilla bean comes from an orchid. There are over 100 species of vanilla orchids in the world, but only three main species are cultivated for vanilla production. Most of our vanilla come from *Vanilla planifolia*. The spanish word, vaina or vainilla means little sheath.

This vine orchid is native to Mexico, where it's been used medicinally for hundreds, if not thousands of years. As far as we know, the Totonaco were the first peoples to harvest vanilla. They were conquered by the Aztecs who demanded this exotic fruit.

In 1528, Montezuma introduced Spanish conquistador Hernan Cortes to the "Drink of the Gods". Cortes returned to Spain bringing Xocolatl, or cocoa, and vanilla with him. For hundreds of years vanilla was a highly sought spice in Europe, only affordable by royalty.

After the Europeans discovered vanilla, they tried desperately to grow it themselves but were unsuccessful for over three hundred years. Then in 1836, botanist Charles Francois Antoine Morren noticed that after bees pollinated the vanilla orchid, the fruit would appear several days later. He began to experiment with hand pollinating the flowers himself; thus, vanilla began cultivating outside of Mexico.

Today, vanilla is still hand pollinated using a technique developed in 1841 by Edmon Albius, a 12 year old slave who lived on the island of Reunion.

Vanilla is so incredibly expensive because of the enormous amount of time and care that goes into every bean pod.

Each orchid flower produces one vanilla bean pod after it's been pollinated by the Melipone bee. The orchid flowers only bloom for one day so timing is everything!

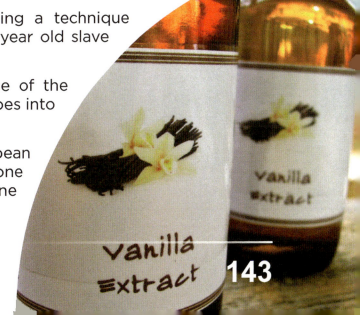

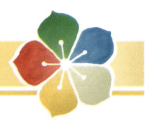

Once a flower has been pollinated, the bean pod will take around 10 months to mature. It has to be harvested at the right time to ensure the highest quality. After the vanilla bean pod is harvested, it goes through an extensive curing process.

> *"Not many herbalists use vanilla medicinally today, probably due to the high cost of the beans. Historically vanilla may have been used as an aphrodesiac, for stomach pain, cough, as a stimulating nervine, for stomach pains and even for venomous bites."*
>
> Kiva Rose
> Herbalist

WHAT YOU'LL NEED...

- At least 12 vanilla beans, possibly more if giving as a gift
- 2 cups of vodka
- pint jar

Begin by cutting the vanilla beans in half.

Place all of the vanilla beans in the pint jar

Cover them with the vodka

Let it sit for 4-6 weeks. After this time, taste the extract to see if the taste is strong enough.

The vanilla beans can stay in the mixture indefinitely. I've heard recommendations that you can keep refilling the jar with vodka after it's 1/4 empty.

Another fun thing to try is to place the vanilla beans in a jar of sugar. The sugar will be left with a vanilla taste.

If you are giving this as a gift, I recommend straining off the vanilla pods and putting the extract in an amber bottle with a new vanilla pod.

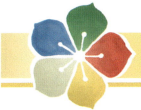

EXERCISE, ADAPTOGEN

Adaptogen Bon Bons

Adaptogen herbs are defined as non-toxic substances that help the body adapt to stressful situations while also normalizing our physiological states.

Of course, adaptogen herbs don't take away stress, but they can improve our response to stress. Most adaptogens are gentle and nourishing, which can be taken long term for best results.

Many herbalists use teas and tinctures as a way of taking herbs. The following recipe explores another traditional use of herbal medicine by mixing powdered herbs into a paste that can be eaten.

But first, let's explore the herbs we'll be using today.

Ashwaganda *(Withania somnifera)*: This herb comes to us from India (also called Indian Ginseng). It's a wonderful restorative tonic especially suitable for people experiencing nervous exhaustion that manifests as insomnia. This herb is a slightly warming and gentle yang tonic.

Shatavari *(Asparagus racemosus)*: Another Indian herb that restores a person's energy level from a worn out and fatigued state. Often used in cases of female or male infertility, this adaptogen is very nutritive. It's considered an immune system tonic, also.

Eleuthero *(Eleutherococcus senticosus)*: This herb was also recently called Siberian Ginseng. It's a gentle adaptogen that's appropriate for most people. David Winston reports that he uses it for people who "work hard, play hard, and hardly sleep." Like other adaptogens, eleuthero supports the immune system and can be taken for extended periods of time.

Licorice *(Glycyrrhiza glabra)*: This sweet-tasting root may be the most commonly used herb in China as it's often added to formulas as a balancer. Licorice has a multitude of uses including soothing dry spasmodic coughs, aiding digestive ulcerations, and healing cold sores. As an adaptogen it regulates the immune system, improves energy levels, and restores balance to the body. It should not be used long term or in large dosages for people with hypertension.

WHAT YOU'LL NEED...

- 1 cup of tahini (sesame paste)
- 1/3 cup of almond butter
- 1/2 cup of honey
- 1/2 cup of chopped almonds
- 1/2 cup of ashwaganda powder
- 1/2 cup of shatavari powder

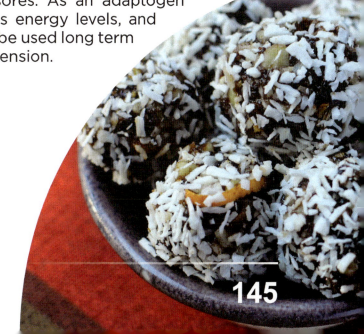

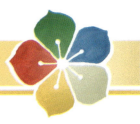

- 1/2 cup of eleuthero powder
- 1/4 cup of licorice powder
- 1 teaspoon of cinnamon
- 1/2 teaspoon of nutmeg
- 1/2 teaspoon of cardamom
- fresh orange zest
- 1/2 cup of cocoa nibs (can substitute chopped chocolate chips if necessary)
- 1 cup of shredded coconut

Begin by mixing all the powdered herbs together. Set them aside once they are combined well.

Over low heat, gently warm the nut butters and honey, stirring constantly. The goal of this isn't to cook the mixture but rather to warm it just enough to help mix it together.

Once it has warmed enough to form a consistent mixture, remove from heat. Immediately stir in the chopped almonds followed by the herbal powder mixture. The end result should be a soft and pliable dough mixture.

After the paste has cooled down, add the cocoa nibs. If added too soon the heat from the mixture could melt them.

After everything is combined, form about a tablespoon of the dough into a ball. You can then roll this ball in a bed of coconut and orange zest.

These balls can be stored in an airtight container in the fridge. In our house, we eat one to three a day.

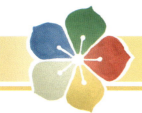

EXERCISE, ADAPTOGEN
Congee

Congee is a comfort food from Asia that can be deeply nourishing.

There are countless recipes out there for congee. The basic recipe is 1 cup rice to 10 cups broth. From there, you can add different nourishing herbs, veggies, and meats. It can be made into a sweet dish by using water and fruits (dried or fresh).

Jujube dates are a wonderfully nourishing fruit common in Chinese herbalism and cooking. I buy jujube dates each fall from this farm located in New Mexico. If you can't find jujube dates, simply omit them from the recipe. Note that jujubes have a pit.

The astragalus roots and reishi slices will not be edible and will need to be removed.

WHAT YOU'LL NEED...

- 1 cup rice
- 10 cups chicken or vegetable broth
- a handful of astragalus root
- 1-2 slices of dried reishi mushroom
- a handful of jujube dates (optional)
- 2 tablespoons of minced garlic
- 2 tablespoons of minced ginger root
- 1 tablespoon of freshly ground black pepper
- 3 pounds of cooked chicken cut into serving pieces
- salt to taste
- scallions (garnish)

Place the rice, broth, and herbs in a large pot. Bring to a boil then immediately reduce to a simmer.

Simmer for an hour stirring occasionally. Add the chicken and simmer for another 1/2 hour stirring frequently. The end consistency should resemble oatmeal. Add more broth if necessary.

Garnish with scallion.

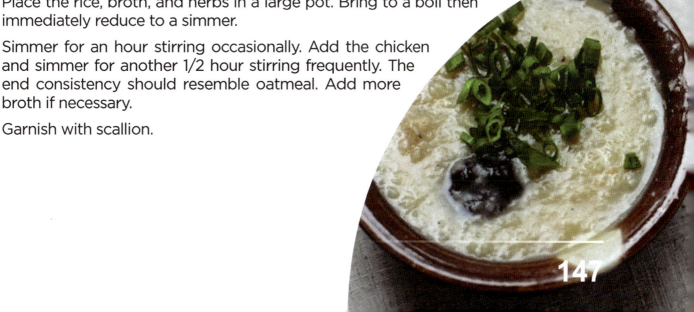

EXERCISE, BLOOD AND YIN TONICS

Blood Building Syrup

All systems of traditional medicine make extensive use of the medicinal properties of both fresh and dried fruit that's cooked with water to make a compote or prepared as medicinal jams and syrups. Ayurveda maintains a large class of medicinal jams called lehyas, which means "to lick." This refers to the method of administration. While they aren't exactly like deserts, compotes, jams, and syrups are a very pleasant way to get the medicine down. Particularly, they're suited to both vata and pitta conditions. The following 'Blood Building Syrup' is an excellent preparation to build up the blood in anemia, infertility, exhaustion, immunodeficiency, or when recovering from chronic disease, medical treatments (e.g. chemotherapy), or surgery. Although it's prepared as a syrup in this recipe, prepare it as a compote. Simply stew the fruit with the herbs and serve it without processing it further.

WHAT YOU'LL NEED...

- 1/2 cup chopped dried figs
- 1/2 cup dried goji berries
- 1/2 cup dried prunes
- 1/2 cup Chinese red dates
- 1 ounce shatavari root (tien men dong or asparagus root)
- 1 ounce cured rehmannia (shu di huang)
- 1 ounce astragalus root (huang qi)
- 1 ounce American ginseng (xi yang shen)
- 2 quarts (4 liters) water
- 2-3 tablespoons ghee
- 2 tablespoons pippali powder
- 1 teaspoon cardamom powder
- 1 teaspoon cinnamon powder
- 1/2 teaspoon clove powder
- 1/4 teaspoon pink salt
- 1 cup organic molasses (approximately)

Directions

Add the dried fruit and herbs (shatavari, rehmannia, astragalus, American ginseng) into a pot along with 2 quarts of water. Bring to a boil and simmer until it is reduced to a syrup-like consistency and the fruit and herbs are squishy (takes about 1 hour).

Allow the fruit-herb decoction to cool and mix in a blender until smooth. Strain the liquid through a mesh strainer into a measuring cup, taking note of exactly how much liquid you are left with. In a separate pan, melt the ghee on medium heat and add the pippali, cardamom, cinnamon, clove, and pink salt.

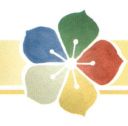

Cook for a minute and add the fruit-herb decoction to this along with an equal part of molasses. Cook on low heat for about 10-15 minutes, stirring frequently. Pour into a clean, dry glass bottle. Seal and store it in a cool location.

The dosage is 1-2 tablespoons twice daily with warm water.

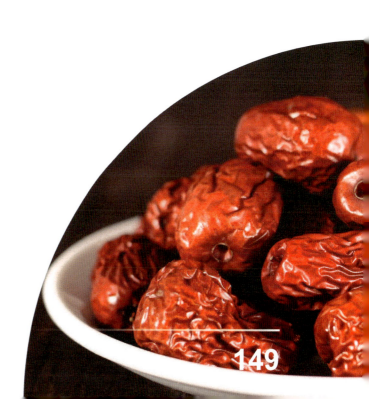

EXERCISE, BLOOD AND YIN TONICS

Borscht

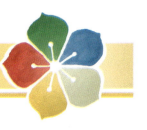

Beet roots are an incredible food and have long been used to support liver health and to build blood.

According to Jo Robinson, author of Eating on the Wild Side, beets are some of the highest antioxidant foods and have nine times more antioxidants than tomatoes; and fifty times more antioxidants than carrots! Beets' unique combination of phytonutrients and antioxidants have been shown to be especially helpful in reducing chronic inflammation.

Beets have a special pigment, betalin, which strongly supports the body's phase 2 detoxification process. Phase 2 detoxification is when the body neutralizes and removes potentially harmful substances from the body by making them water soluble.

There are lots of different borscht recipes out there. In this version, I included those incredibly nutritious beet greens and added extra pepper for zing and increased nutrient absorption.

WHAT YOU'LL NEED...

- 1 & 1/2 cups cubed potatoes
- 2 cups cubed beets
- 6 cups chicken or vegetable broth
- 2 tablespoons butter
- 1 1/2 cups chopped onions
- 4 garlic cloves minced
- 1 cup chopped beet greens
- 1 teaspoon caraway seeds
- 2 teaspoons salt (or to taste)
- 1 celery stalk, chopped
- 1 large carrot, sliced
- 3 cups coarsely chopped purple cabbage
- 2-3 tablespoons freshly ground black pepper
- 2 bay leaves
- 1 tablespoon balsamic vinegar
- 1 tablespoon honey
- 1 cup tomato puree
- sour cream (optional)
- green onions for garnish

Heat the butter in a large pot. Sauté the onions until they are translucent.

Add the garlic, caraway seeds, salt, pepper, and bay leaves. Sauté for 1 minute.

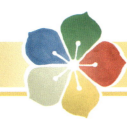

Add the celery, carrots, cabbage, beets, potatoes, mushrooms, and stock. Simmer until all the vegetables are tender (takes about 30 minutes).

Stir in the balsamic vinegar, beet greens, honey, and tomato puree. Cover and simmer for 5 more minutes.

Serve with a dollop of sour cream (optional) and green onions for garnish.

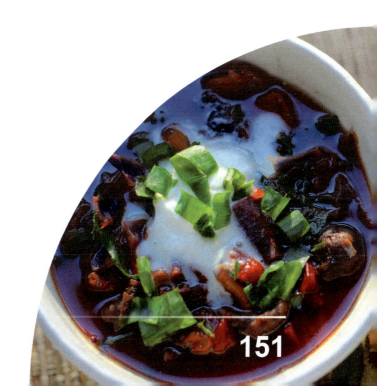

EXERCISE, BLOOD AND YIN TONICS
Yellow Dock Syrup

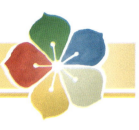

Yellow dock syrup is a traditional western herbal formula that is used to build blood. Yellow dock root helps the body utilize iron and the black strap of molasses contains iron. Dong quai is another classic blood building herb and goji berries are specific for building liver blood.

For a simpler syrup, you can omit the dong quai and goji berries and use the yellow dock syrup and the blackstrap molasses.

WHAT YOU'LL NEED...

- 1 ounce dried or fresh yellow dock root
- 1 ounce dried dong quai
- 1 ounce dried goji berries
- enough water to cover the herbs by two inches
- black strap molasses

Place the herbs and water in a medium sized pan.

Simmer for 40 minutes or until it is reduced by half.

Strain and measure the liquid.

Add an equal part of black strap molasses to the liquid.

Store it in the fridge. Take 1-2 tablespoons in divided doses throughout the day.

Yellow dock is a mild laxative. If you develop loose stools while using this, use a lower dose. This recipe may not be the best choice for someone who already has loose stools.

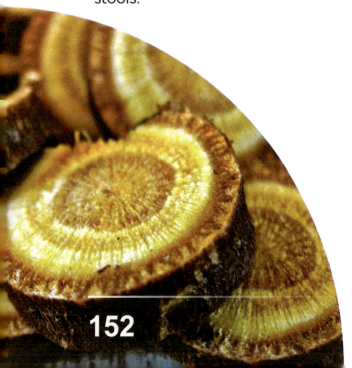

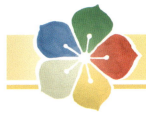

EXERCISE, DEMULCENT

Marshmallow Infusion

I love single herbs that seemingly do everything. Their complexity could inspire a lifetime of devotion to learning the intricate ways they could be used for food and medicine. The ways they support their habitat and the gifts they bring the earth are astonishing. Single herbs that can be used in a variety of ways are called polycrest herbs.

At first glance marshmallow seems like a specific plant. Its claim to fame is being the #1 go-to demulcent herb for many herbalists.

Demulcent herbs are slimy and thick. They're typically used to soothe mucous membranes. Like many demulcent herbs, marshmallow is cooling and moistening, which brings relief to hot and dry conditions.

Despite having the specificity of being a demulcent herb, marshmallow is a polycrest herb. It's been used for centuries in a broad range of ways. The genus name for marshmallow is derived from the Greek word altho, which means "to cure." This gives us a powerful indication of how highly regarded this plant was in ancient times.

The majority of the time, we make teas and long infusions. We use hot water to extract the plant material, but marshmallow roots are typically prepared using cold water.

Marshmallow roots are high in polysaccharides and starches. By using a cold infusion, you extract mainly the mucilaginous polysaccharides. If you simmer the root you also extract the starches in the plant (which is okay—the cold infusion is considered to be a purer extract of the mucilage.)

WHAT YOU'LL NEED...

- a jar and lid
- marshmallow root
- lukewarm water
- time

To make this preparation, simply fill a jar 1/4 of the way with marshmallow root.

Then fill the jar with lukewarm water and cover it with a lid.

Let it sit for a minimum of 4 hours or overnight. The water should change color to a soft yellow.

Strain off the roots. The resulting liquid should be thick and viscous.

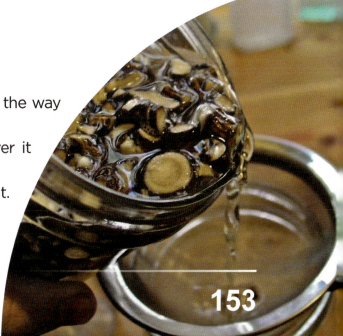

EXERCISE, DEMULCENT

Sore Throat Pastilles

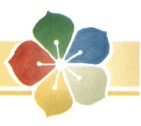

Pastilles are a fancy name for herbal pills. They can be made simply by combining powdered herbs with a liquid to form a type of dough. They can be made in advance or made when needed.

I really like using herb powders as part of my herbal creations - in this way we are consuming the whole herb and not just extracting certain parts of the herb with water, alcohol, or vinegar.

Powdered herbs will lose their potency faster than herbs stored in their whole form, so be sure to use recently powdered herbs by getting them from a reputable apothecary or by powdering them yourself.

Before getting started on the recipe, let's take a look at sore throats. Why we are using these particular herbs for sore throats?

When throats are sore due to symptoms of a cold or flu, they're usually red, hot, scratchy, swollen, and downright uncomfortable. To help relieve the discomfort, we can use cooling, demulcent, and astringent herbs.

Cooling herbs bring relief to a hot and red throat. Demulcent herbs can soothe a dry irritated throat, and astringent herbs can tighten and tone swollen tissues in the throat.

By understanding the state of the tissues involved and by understanding how to match those with herbs, we can be more effective at matching herbs and people.

Here's a closer look at the herbs in this recipe.

Rose Petals *(Rosa spp.)*

Cooling and astringent, rose can reduce inflammation and relieve pain. All parts of the rose are astringent and can be used in a variety of ways. Using the petals in medicine adds a sense of luxury.

Sage leaves *(Salvia officinalis)*

Most of us use this pungent spice once or twice a year when making stuffing to accompany the turkey, but sage offers us many healing attributes. It's antimicrobial and astringent, meaning that it can disable pathogens on contact while tightening and toning tissues. It has a long history of use for mouth ulcerations and sore throats.

Marshmallow *(Althaea officinalis)*

This sweet and demulcent herb can boost our immune system, relieve a dry cough,

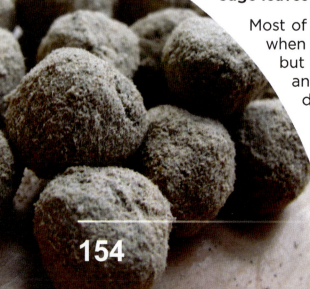

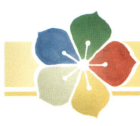

and soothe a sore, irritated throat. Common mallow (*Malva neglecta*) can be used similarly and it probably grows somewhere near you.

Honey

Honey is wonderfully soothing for sore throats and it's also antimicrobial. I like to use raw local honey. Bee keepers are springing up all over the US, making this a fairly easy product to find.

Today's recipe is a favorite in our house. I learned of it years ago from herbalist Kiva Rose.

WHAT YOU'LL NEED...

- 1 tablespoon powdered rose petals
- 1/2 tablespoon powdered sage leaves
- 2 tablespoons of marshmallow root
- 1 1/2 tablespoons of warmed honey
- *optional: additional cinnamon and rose powders*

Mix the powdered herbs together.

Warm some honey over really low heat. We want this honey to be warm enough to have a syrup consistency but never hot.

Add the honey slowly to the powdered herbs. I like to add a little honey, stir, and reevaluate for the consistency. The end result should be a soft doughy mixture that is not too sticky. You can adjust the honey and powder as necessary.

Once you have mixed the herbs and honey together, you can roll them into balls.

I like to finish the pastilles by rolling them in some additional rose petal and cinnamon powder.

These can be used immediately or stored in the fridge for a couple of weeks.

Besides being great for sore throats, pastilles can be used for a variety of other situations as well. Remember, they are cooling and soothing making them great for hot digestive problems like ulcers and heartburn.

I've used similar formulas for people experiencing hot flashes and night sweats.

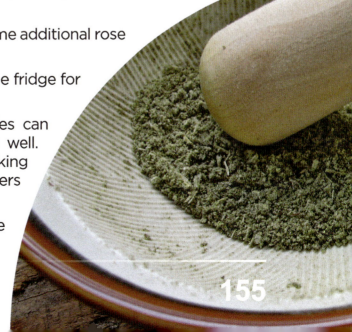

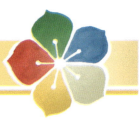

Once you understand the basic concept of making herbal pastilles, you'll see there are many variations. The herbs you use can vary as well as the liquid that holds them together.

I generally like to use a demulcent herb like marshmallow or slippery elm as a base when making pastilles as this creates a nice texture.

You can substitute maple syrup for the honey or use a tea as the liquid. When using water as the liquid to hold them together, you either need to consume them quickly or dry them out completely before storing.

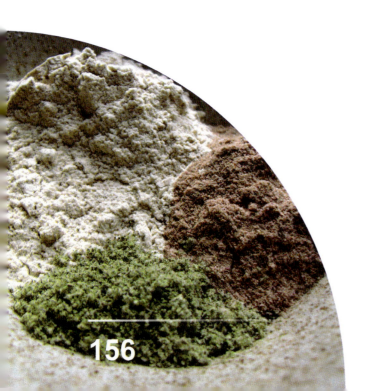

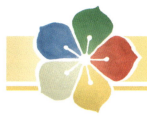

EXERCISE, IMMUNOMODULATING

Nourishing Bone Broth

Bone broth stock is both the secret of delicious soups and a wonderful way to get immunomodulating herbs as food.

It's high in calcium, magnesium, phosphorus, silicon, sulphur, trace minerals, chondroitin sulphates, and glucosamine. Boiling the bones releases gelatin into the broth (which is why it hardens slightly when cooled).

This recipe is more of a general guideline as there are many ways to make bone broth soup. This can also be made in whatever quantity you like. I like to make big batches and freeze what I don't need immediately.

I fill a pan about 1/3 of the way with bones, then add in the herbs and vegetables, and finally fill the pot with water.

This broth can then be the base for soups or can simply be drank as is, perhaps with a bit of miso added to it. Yum!

WHAT YOU'LL NEED...

- several bones from poultry or beef (preferably bones that have marrow)
- 1 tablespoon apple cider vinegar (it helps to draw out the calcium from the bones)
- 1 onion coarsely chopped (skin too)
- 2 carrots coarsely chopped
- 1 big handful of dried stinging nettle leaf
- several dandelion roots coarsely chopped or a handful of dried root
- a couple large handfuls of sliced dried astragalus root
- 2 celery ribs coarsely chopped (or any other vegetable scraps)
- water to fill the pot

Place everything in a large pot except for the handful of aromatic herbs.

Fill the pot with water and bring to a boil slowly.

Once it is boiling, reduce to a simmer.

After awhile, you will see some foam forming at the top. Gently skim this off every couple of minutes until the broth runs clear.

When ready, strain off all materials and discard.

Store the broth in the fridge or freezer until ready to use for soups, roasts, chili, etc.

This can also be cooked in a crock pot.

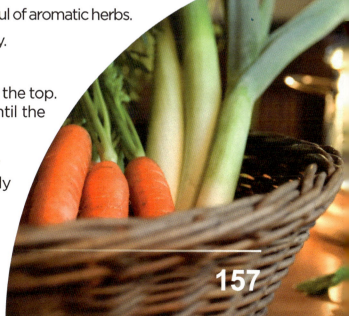

EXERCISE, IMMUNOMODULATING

Shitake Shallot Butter

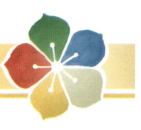

We like to serve this butter warmed on bread for our dinner guests. We are always asked for the recipe. It's savory and delicious.

WHAT YOU'LL NEED...

- 1 stick of butter
- 1-2 shitake mushrooms (can use white button mushrooms, too)
- 1 small shallot

Begin by placing the stick of butter in a warm place in order to soften it.

Next, mince the mushroom(s) and shallot.

Once the butter is softened, mix in the minced mushroom and shallot.

For Shitake and Shallot Bread (consider this a fancy garlic bread)

Since all mushrooms should be cooked prior to eating, we like to spread this herbal butter onto loaves of bread and heat thoroughly in the oven.

To do this:
1. Take a whole loaf of bread and cut it into slices, leaving the bottom crust still attached (so it's not cut all the way through).
2. Spread a generous portion of the herbed butter on each slice of bread.
3. Place it in a casserole container with a lid or wrap in aluminum foil.
4. Bake for 20 minutes or until the butter is melted through.
5. Serve while warm.

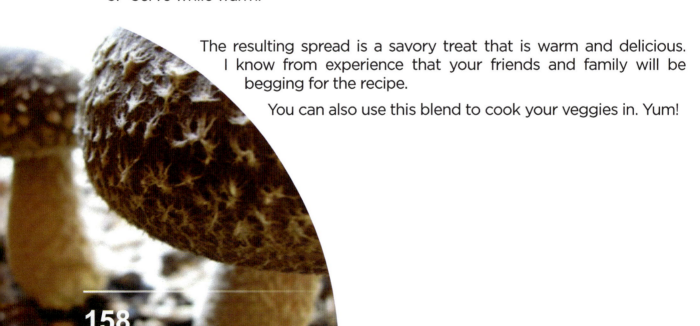

The resulting spread is a savory treat that is warm and delicious. I know from experience that your friends and family will be begging for the recipe.

You can also use this blend to cook your veggies in. Yum!

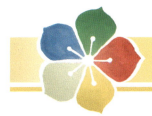

EXERCISE, VULNERARY

Comfrey Poultice

Comfrey is an amazing vulnerary herb. It can knit together wounds so fast you'd almost swear you could watch it happen before your eyes.

Comfrey is so good at healing wounds that you have to be careful not to apply comfrey to infected wounds since it can seal the infection in, causing serious problems.

Comfrey is also great for healing broken bones. Again, it's so good at this that it's cautioned not to use comfrey on a broken bone unless the bone has been set. Otherwise, it could heal the bones out of place.

Pretty amazing plant!

Here are directions on how to make your own basic comfrey leaf poultice.

WHAT YOU'LL NEED...

- several large fresh comfrey leaves
- an old t-shirt or cheesecloth
- masking tape (or something else like vet wrap to hold it in place)

Begin by chopping up the comfrey leaves. They can be a bit pokey, so you may want to wear gloves. Mince them well.

Using a mortar and pestle (or simply using a sturdy wooden spoon in a bowl), mash the comfrey leaves until they form a paste. You can also put them in a blender or food processor.

You want to end up with a paste of comfrey leaves.

Place this over the desired area. Wrap an old t-shirt or something similar around the poultice. Secure it with tape.

This can be changed up to three times a day.

To freeze comfrey poultices for later use, make the comfrey paste and then put it in a ziplock or tupperware in the freezer. Refresh each growing season.

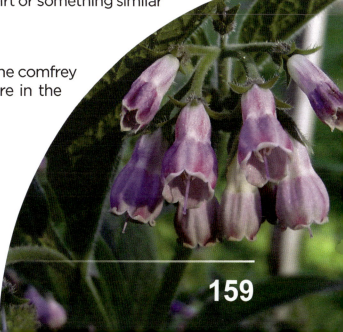

EXERCISE, VULNERARY
Plantain Salve

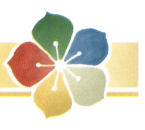

This exercise is a multi-part process to create your own vulnerary healing salve. This recipe is perfect for minor cuts and scrapes.

Plantain is best when fresh or just barely dried. Using fresh plantain in an oil infusion is a bit tricky because introducing water to oil can make it mold. This recipe will be best if you are able to harvest plantain yourself and dry it; or even just allowing it to wilt overnight to remove most of the water content.

If you aren't able to harvest your own plantain, then it can also be bought dried from your local herbal apothecary or favorite online retailer.

WHAT YOU'LL NEED...

- freshly dried plantain (just wilted overnight is even better)
- dried calendula flowers
- dried lavender flowers
- jar
- olive oil
- beeswax
- small jars
- lavender essential oil (optional)

Step 1: Preparing the Essentials

You can use any size jar you would like for this. Simply fill the jar halfway with equal parts of plantain, calendula, and lavender flowers.

Then, fill the jar completely with olive oil. Stir well. Put a lid on it.

Let this sit in a cool area for 6 weeks. Open up the jar and stir it a couple times a week.

After 6 weeks strain the herbs from the oil. Compost the herbs and save the oil.

Step 2: Making a Salve

Now that you have your herbal infused oil, you can make your salve.

I use 1 ounce of beeswax for every cup of oil. So let's say you're going to make a salve using one cup of oil.

Place the beeswax in a double boiler and gently melt it. Once it's entirely melted stir in the oil. Stir with a popsicle stick until it is melted and combined. Remove from heat.

If desired, add 20-40 drops of lavender essential oil. Stir well.

Pour immediately into small jars. Label and use within a year.

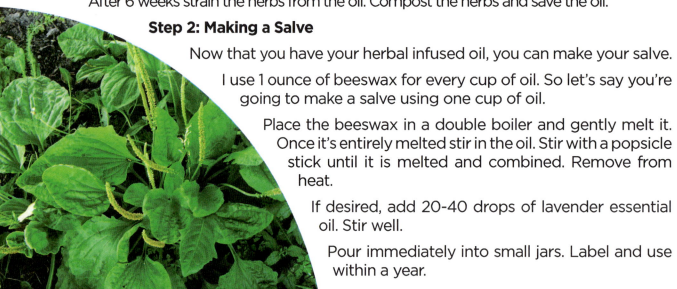

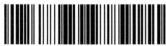

Made in the USA
Charleston, SC
11 November 2015